Empirical Likelihood Method in Survival Analysis

Chapman & Hall/CRC Biostatistics Series

Published Titles

Adaptive Design Methods in Clinical Trials, Second Edition
Shein-Chung Chow and Mark Chang

Adaptive Designs for Sequential Treatment Allocation
Alessandro Baldi Antognini and Alessandra Giovagnoli

Adaptive Design Theory and Implementation Using SAS and R, Second Edition
Mark Chang

Advanced Bayesian Methods for Medical Test Accuracy
Lyle D. Broemeling

Advances in Clinical Trial Biostatistics
Nancy L. Geller

Applied Meta-Analysis with R
Ding-Geng (Din) Chen and Karl E. Peace

Basic Statistics and Pharmaceutical Statistical Applications, Second Edition
James E. De Muth

Bayesian Adaptive Methods for Clinical Trials
Scott M. Berry, Bradley P. Carlin, J. Jack Lee, and Peter Muller

Bayesian Analysis Made Simple: An Excel GUI for WinBUGS
Phil Woodward

Bayesian Methods for Measures of Agreement
Lyle D. Broemeling

Bayesian Methods in Epidemiology
Lyle D. Broemeling

Bayesian Methods in Health Economics
Gianluca Baio

Bayesian Missing Data Problems: EM, Data Augmentation and Noniterative Computation
Ming T. Tan, Guo-Liang Tian, and Kai Wang Ng

Bayesian Modeling in Bioinformatics
Dipak K. Dey, Samiran Ghosh, and Bani K. Mallick

Benefit-Risk Assessment in Pharmaceutical Research and Development
Andreas Sashegyi, James Felli, and Rebecca Noel

Biosimilars: Design and Analysis of Follow-on Biologics
Shein-Chung Chow

Biostatistics: A Computing Approach
Stewart J. Anderson

Causal Analysis in Biomedicine and Epidemiology: Based on Minimal Sufficient Causation
Mikel Aickin

Clinical and Statistical Considerations in Personalized Medicine
Claudio Carini, Sandeep Menon, and Mark Chang

Clinical Trial Data Analysis using R
Ding-Geng (Din) Chen and Karl E. Peace

Clinical Trial Methodology
Karl E. Peace and Ding-Geng (Din) Chen

Computational Methods in Biomedical Research
Ravindra Khattree and Dayanand N. Naik

Computational Pharmacokinetics
Anders Källén

Confidence Intervals for Proportions and Related Measures of Effect Size
Robert G. Newcombe

Controversial Statistical Issues in Clinical Trials
Shein-Chung Chow

Data and Safety Monitoring Committees in Clinical Trials
Jay Herson

Design and Analysis of Animal Studies in Pharmaceutical Development
Shein-Chung Chow and Jen-pei Liu

Design and Analysis of Bioavailability and Bioequivalence Studies, Third Edition
Shein-Chung Chow and Jen-pei Liu

Design and Analysis of Bridging Studies
Jen-pei Liu, Shein-Chung Chow, and Chin-Fu Hsiao

Design and Analysis of Clinical Trials for Predictive Medicine
Shigeyuki Matsui, Marc Buyse, and Richard Simon

Design and Analysis of Clinical Trials with Time-to-Event Endpoints
Karl E. Peace

Design and Analysis of Non-Inferiority Trials
Mark D. Rothmann, Brian L. Wiens, and Ivan S. F. Chan

Difference Equations with Public Health Applications
Lemuel A. Moyé and Asha Seth Kapadia

DNA Methylation Microarrays: Experimental Design and Statistical Analysis
Sun-Chong Wang and Arturas Petronis

DNA Microarrays and Related Genomics Techniques: Design, Analysis, and Interpretation of Experiments
David B. Allison, Grier P. Page, T. Mark Beasley, and Jode W. Edwards

Dose Finding by the Continual Reassessment Method
Ying Kuen Cheung

Elementary Bayesian Biostatistics
Lemuel A. Moyé

Empirical Likelihood Method in Survival Analysis
Mai Zhou

Frailty Models in Survival Analysis
Andreas Wienke

Generalized Linear Models: A Bayesian Perspective
Dipak K. Dey, Sujit K. Ghosh, and Bani K. Mallick

Handbook of Regression and Modeling: Applications for the Clinical and Pharmaceutical Industries
Daryl S. Paulson

Inference Principles for Biostatisticians
Ian C. Marschner

Interval-Censored Time-to-Event Data: Methods and Applications
Ding-Geng (Din) Chen, Jianguo Sun, and Karl E. Peace

Introductory Adaptive Trial Designs: A Practical Guide with R
Mark Chang

Joint Models for Longitudinal and Time-to-Event Data: With Applications in R
Dimitris Rizopoulos

Measures of Interobserver Agreement and Reliability, Second Edition
Mohamed M. Shoukri

Medical Biostatistics, Third Edition
A. Indrayan

Meta-Analysis in Medicine and Health Policy
Dalene Stangl and Donald A. Berry

Chapman & Hall/CRC Biostatistics Series

Empirical Likelihood Method in Survival Analysis

Mai Zhou

University of Kentucky

Lexington, USA

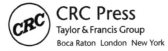

CRC Press is an imprint of the
Taylor & Francis Group, an **informa** business

A CHAPMAN & HALL BOOK

CRC Press
Taylor & Francis Group
6000 Broken Sound Parkway NW, Suite 300
Boca Raton, FL 33487-2742

First issued in paperback 2019

© 2016 by Taylor & Francis Group, LLC
CRC Press is an imprint of Taylor & Francis Group, an Informa business

No claim to original U.S. Government works

ISBN-13: 978-1-4665-5492-4 (hbk)
ISBN-13: 978-0-367-37757-1 (pbk)

**Visit the Taylor & Francis Web site at
http://www.taylorandfrancis.com**

**and the CRC Press Web site at
http://www.crcpress.com**

Contents

CONTENTS

List of Figures

List of Tables

Preface

The first book on empirical likelihood was published in 2001 (by Owen and also from CRC), thirteen years after Owen published his first paper on empirical likelihood in 1988 [78].

This fascinating methodology attracted a lot of researchers and has been under rapid development ever since. Numerous papers have been published since then and the list is getting longer every day.

It is now fourteen years since the publication of Owen's 2001 book on empirical likelihood. I feel the time is perhaps ripe for another book on empirical likelihood.

Aside from the obvious accumulation of research progress in the fourteen years since, another obvious development is the vastly improved computing power and universal availability of computers. No longer are expensive workstations in the labs available only to a few. They are everywhere and in every student's backpack.

During the last 14 years, the software R became the most popular choice of language among statistics researchers, and went from version 1.x.x to 3.x.x. I feel the easy-to-use, widely available R software for calculating empirical likelihood will boost the everyday use of empirical likelihood and in turn stimulate more research in this area.

This book includes many worked out examples with the associated R code. You can copy and paste them into an R command window.

The R packages used in this book include `emplik`, `survival`, KMsurv, ELYP. We also briefly mention related packages `km.ci`, `kmc`, `gmm`, `rms`, `el.convex`. The latter group of packages is not crucial when reading this book. The package `emplik` is version 1.01 at the time of writing this book. This package has over 12 years of history. On the other hand, the package ELYP is less refined and is version 0.72.

We use the `survival` package for both its datasets and some of the estimation functions (for example, to obtain the Cox partial likelihood estimate). The package KMsurv contains only datasets, and we use them in several examples. The package `emplik` is the main package for calculations related to empirical likelihood, except for those related to the Cox model, which are in the package ELYP. The package kmc contains the functions that implement the recursive algorithm we describe in Chapter 6. It is still quite fluid and should eventually be integrated into `emplik` in the future. Finally, the package `km.ci` provides empirical likelihood confidence intervals and confidence bands for the Kaplan–Meier survival probabilities.

I will keep updating and uploading the package `emplik` and ELYP to the public

xvi   PREFACE

repository CRAN after the publication of the book, and maintain a Web page for any updates:

```
http://www.ms.uky.edu/~mai/EmpLik.html
```

The empirical likelihood method has its root in survival analysis. The very first paper originating the empirical likelihood method [112] is about empirical likelihood with the Kaplan–Meier estimator. So it seems to me that the empirical likelihood method naturally fits in with survival analysis. Also, over the years I have worked mostly on the empirical likelihood applications in survival analysis. So I chose to concentrate on this area.

Owen [81] covers much wider topics and also contains several sections about empirical likelihood with various censored, truncated, or other incomplete data. He discussed many forms of censoring, including interval censoring and double censoring. This book deals only with right censored data. Also, we do not discuss high-order asymptotic results for the empirical likelihood ratio. I feel the practical usefulness of high-order results in survival analysis concerning empirical likelihood ratio is not clear at this moment.

The core content of the book is Chapters 1, 2, 3, 4 (less Section 4.5), and 6. Chapter 1 discuss the empirical likelihood for right censored data, Chapter 6 for some computational tricks for censored data empirical likelihood, and the rest of the materials are pretty much standard survival analysis topics, treated with empirical likelihood. Basic knowledge of survival analysis is assumed.

Chapter 5 covers semi-parametric accelerated failure time models. This subject has a long history, but somehow standard software does not usually include this model and it is less used in practice (compared to the Cox regression model).

Section 4.5 discusses a recent extension of the Cox model by Yang and Prentice [129]. I include it here because I believe the empirical likelihood method is particularly suited for the statistical inference of this model.

Chapter 7 is about the optimality of confidence regions derived from empirical likelihood ratio tests or plug-in empirical likelihood ratio tests. It is a bit of a surprise that confidence regions can be so different in shape and orientation based on censored data. Chapter 8 collects mainly several empirical likelihood confidence band results, among other things.

There is a long list of people to whom I want to say THANK YOU. I am afraid the list is so long that I won't be able to stop for a long time. So instead of all the names, I shall list several categories.

First, all my colleagues. I have benefited tremendously over the years by reading your work and writings, by personal interactions, and in some cases, by collaborating on research. Some of the names appear in the reference list at the end of this book, but there are many more whose names do not appear in the references. THANK YOU!

I am also grateful to my students. I enjoyed working with you all.

I also want to acknowledge the support of an NSF grant.

I want to thank the many people who helped me put together this manuscript, correcting numerous typos and awkward grammar. All the remaining errors are my own.

Finally, I want to thank my family; they helped in this book project in numerous ways.

Mai Zhou

Chapter 1

Introduction

Survival analysis has long been a classic area of statistical study. For example, the famous Kaplan–Meier estimator got its name from a paper published in the year 1958. Many textbooks on survival analysis are available and the list is still growing. The main survival analysis procedures are available in all major statistical software packages. On the other hand, empirical likelihood is a methodology that has only recently been developed. The name "empirical likelihood" seems to appear first in Owen's 1988 paper. Only one book so far is available on empirical likelihood and most commercial statistical software does not yet include empirical likelihood procedures.

1.1 Survival Analysis

What is survival analysis? One might say "survival analysis is the statistical analysis of failure time data." In fact, some books are titled exactly as such. It is certainly correct, but it begs people to ask "what is failure time data?," which then takes longer to explain.

One might also say that "survival analysis is Kaplan–Meier estimator + log-rank test + Cox proportional hazards model." This description is too simplistic, but certainly very specific and constructive.

Perhaps we should be asking: what is the difference between survival analysis and regular statistical analysis? Or what are the unique features of survival analysis not seen in other branches of statistics?

We can list several features unique to survival analysis:

1. In survival analysis, the parameters of interest are often the "hazard" instead of cumulative distribution function (CDF) or mean.

2. In survival analysis, the available data is subject to censoring.

3. In survival analysis, nonparametric procedures are more common.

Empirical likelihood is a nonparametric method and thus fits into the third point above for survival analysis. We also point out that the Kaplan–Meier estimator, log-rank test and Cox model are all nonparametric procedures. Let us discuss the above features in more detail.

1.1.1   Hazard Function

Let $F(t)$ denote the CDF of the random variable X of interest; then the cumulative hazard function is defined as

$$\Lambda(t) = \int_{-\infty}^{t} \frac{dF(s)}{1 - F(s-)} \, . \tag{1.1}$$

We comment that this definition is valid for either continuous or discrete CDF $F(t)$, and for X that can take negative values. If $F(t)$ is discrete, the integration is the Stieljes integral. When the CDF is continuous, $F(s-) = F(s)$, the integration on the right-hand side can be simplified to $-\log(1 - F(t))$ and thus we have (for the continuous case)

$$\Lambda(t) = -\log(1 - F(t)). \tag{1.2}$$

If the CDF has a density $f(s)$, then

$$\Lambda(t) = \int_{-\infty}^{t} \frac{f(s)}{1 - F(s)} ds$$

and

$$\frac{\partial}{\partial t} \Lambda(t) = \frac{f(t)}{1 - F(t)} \, .$$

If we define the *hazard function* $h(t)$ as

$$h(t) = \frac{f(t)}{1 - F(t)} \, ,$$

then the relation between $\Lambda(t)$ and $h(t)$ is similar to that of CDF $F(t)$ to the density $f(t)$, i.e., $\Lambda(t) = \int_{-\infty}^{t} h(s) ds$ and $\frac{\partial}{\partial t} \Lambda(t) = h(t)$.

The probabilistic interpretation of hazard $h(t)$ is that $h(t)dt$ is the conditional probability of the random variable taking a value in $[t, t + dt)$, given it is larger than or equal to t:

$$h(t)dt = \frac{f(t)dt}{1 - F(t-)} = P(t \leq X < t + dt | X \geq t) \, .$$

Compare this to the similar interpretation for the density $f(t)$:

$$f(t)dt = P(t \leq X < t + dt) \, .$$

The hazard $h(t)$ must be nonnegative but does not have an upper bound. The cumulative hazard function $\Lambda(t)$ must be nonnegative and nondecreasing, but again can be unbounded. In fact, if the CDF is continuous, then $\Lambda(t)$ must be unbounded. This can be seen from $\Lambda(t) = -\log(1 - F(t))$. On the other hand, if the CDF is discrete, then $\Lambda(t)$ does not increase to infinity as t increases, but the last jump is always of size one. This can be seen by (supposing t^* is the last jump point)

$$\Delta \Lambda(t_{last}) = \Delta \Lambda(t^*) = \frac{\Delta F(t^*)}{1 - F(t^*-)} = 1 \, ,$$

because $\Delta F(t^*) = F(t^*+) - F(t^*-) = 1 - F(t^*-)$.

The inverse formula that recovers the CDF given a cumulative hazard is a bit awkward in the sense that the continuous and discrete versions look quite different: if the CDF/cumulative hazard is continuous, then

$$1 - F(t) = e^{-\Lambda(t)} . \qquad (1.3)$$

If the CDF/cumulative hazard is purely discrete, then we have

$$1 - F(t) = \prod_{s \leq t} (1 - \Delta\Lambda(s)) , \qquad (1.4)$$

where $\Delta\Lambda(s) = \Lambda(s+) - \Lambda(s-)$. We notice that there are at most a countable many terms in the product, because there are at most a countable number of jumps in a monotone function.

In the case of a partly continuous, partly discrete CDF/cumulative hazard, we have to combine the two formulae:

$$1 - F(t) = e^{-\Lambda_c(t)} \prod_{s \leq t} (1 - \Delta\Lambda(s)) \qquad (1.5)$$

where $\Lambda_c(t)$ is the continuous part of the cumulative hazard:

$$\Lambda_c(t) = \Lambda(t) - \sum_{s \leq t} \Delta\Lambda(s) .$$

Our discussion later in this book will mostly focus either on the continuous case or the purely discrete case, not on the mixed case.

The nonparametric estimation of the cumulative hazard function leads to the Nelson–Aalen estimator. The two sample log-rank test can be viewed as comparing the two hazard functions from two samples. The Cox proportional hazards model is a regression model which models how the ratio of hazards relates to the covariates. We shall discuss the Cox model in Chapter 4 and review the Nelson–Aalen estimator and log-rank test in subsections later in the present chapter.

Remark: At first glance, it is not clear how a rather innocent looking transformation of CDF to hazard has such an influence on survival analysis. For one thing, it removed the constraint that the jumps of a CDF must sum to one. Second, by working on conditional probabilities, it localized the parameters and made the estimation problem easier with censoring. This also leads to the application of martingales in survival analysis.

1.1.2   Censored Observations

The random variable of interest in survival analysis is "time to failure," denoted by X. Typically this is a positive, continuous random variable. Between the start and the end of a "life," a lot can happen, and often there are some conditions that prevent us from following up the "life" to its eventual failure. This leads to censoring.

Typically, right censored survival data looks like

$$3+, 6, 2.2, 8+, 12, \cdots$$

where a plus sign means the actual "time to failure" is longer than the recorded time. For example, the first survival time above is somewhat larger than 3.

Censored observations are commonly recorded in software as two vectors instead of a plus:

$$
\begin{aligned}
T &= (3, 6, 2.2, 8, 12, \cdots) \\
\delta &= (0, 1, 1, 0, 1, \cdots)
\end{aligned}
$$

with $(T_1, \delta_1) = (3, 0)$, $(T_2, \delta_2) = (6, 1)$, etc.

The following R code looks at the first few lines of the dataset `veteran` from the `survival` package, and also the usual wrapper for the time and status vectors.

```
library(survival)
data(veteran)
head(veteran)
##    trt celltype time status karno diagtime age prior
## 1    1 squamous   72      1    60        7  69     0
## 2    1 squamous  411      1    70        5  64    10
## 3    1 squamous  228      1    60        3  38     0
## 4    1 squamous  126      1    60        9  63    10
## 5    1 squamous  118      1    70       11  65    10
## 6    1 squamous   10      1    20        5  49     0
Surv(veteran$time,  veteran$status)
##  [1]  72  411  228  126  118   10   82  110  314  100+  42
## [12]   8  144  25+  11   30  384    4   54   13  123+  97+
## ......
```

We further assume for each survival time there is a "follow-up" time, such that the reason that prevents us from observing the entire survival time is due to the follow-up time falling short of the survival time.

Suppose X is the lifetime of interest whose distribution $F(t)$ is of interest. Due to censoring, we only observe the pair T, δ, where

$$T = \min(X, C); \quad \delta = I[X \leq C].$$

The variable C above is the follow-up time, or censoring time. We assume C is independent of X, and has a CDF $G(t)$.

This is called the random independent censorship model.

1.1.3 Parametric and Nonparametric Models

A family of distributions indexed by a finite number of unknown parameters is called a parametric model. Nonparametric models can be viewed as parametric models with *infinitely* many parameters.

In the parametric model setting, the task is often to estimate the unknown parameter. Once we know the value of the parameters, we have a complete picture of the model. In the nonparametric model, the task can be either to estimate a finite dimensional feature of the infinite dimensional parameter or to estimate the infinite dimensional parameter itself.

Example 1 *The family of exponential distributions with unknown parameter $\lambda \in R^+$ is a parametric model with one parameter. We could also specify the model using the hazard function: the exponential family of distributions is all distributions with a constant hazard function:*

$$h(t) = \lambda, \quad for\ t > 0.$$

Example 2 *We can define a piecewise exponential distribution family with k parameters as follows. For a partition of the positive real line $0 = t_0 < t_1 < t_2 < \cdots < t_{k-1} < t_k = \infty$, the piecewise exponential distribution is a distribution with the following hazard function*

$$h(t) = \lambda_i \quad for \quad t_{i-1} \leq t < t_i; \quad i = 1,2,\cdots,k.$$

We assume the partition points, t_i, are given constants and only the $\lambda_i > 0$ are unknown parameters. So there are k unknown parameters.

Example 3 *A nonparametric model can be defined as a family of distributions with arbitrary (thus infinitely dimensional) hazard functions. For reasons that will become apparent later, we would like to define the nonparametric models using the cumulative hazard function $\Lambda(t)$ (or cumulative distribution function). Thus a nonparametric model is the family of all distributions with arbitrary cumulative hazard function $\Lambda(t)$. This way we include the possibility of a distribution with a discrete cumulative hazard function. Notice the cumulative hazard function of Example 2 is continuous.*

1.1.4 Parametric Maximum Likelihood Estimator

The maximum likelihood estimator (MLE) of the parameter(s) in the above parametric Examples 1 and 2 can be obtained by the usual calculations.

Suppose (T_i, δ_i), $i = 1,2,\cdots,n$ is a random sample of right censored lifetimes from the random independent censorship model.

Let us denote the distribution of lifetimes X_i by $F(\cdot)$, and density by $f(\cdot)$. Denote the distribution of the censoring times C_i by $G(\cdot)$.

The parametric likelihood function based on the (T_i, δ_i) is

$$P-lik = \prod_{i=1}^n P(T = t_i, d = \delta_i) = \prod_{\delta_i=1} [(1-G(t_i))f(t_i)dt] \prod_{\delta_i=0} [(1-F(t_i)dG(t_i)].$$

We usually drop the terms that involve censoring distribution G.

Using the relationship between distribution and hazard, or cumulative hazard, the parametric likelihood function can be written as

$$P - lik = \prod_{i=1}^{n} [h(t_i)dt]^{\delta_i} \exp[-\Lambda(t_i)] \, ,$$

where $h(\cdot)$ is the hazard function, and $\Lambda(\cdot)$ is the cumulative hazard function of the lifetimes X_i.

Example 4 *For the exponential model (model 1), we substitute $h(t_i) = \lambda$ and $\Lambda(t_i) = \lambda t_i$ in the above $P - lik$. We can easily find that the (parametric) MLE of λ is*

$$\hat{\lambda} = \frac{\sum_{i=1}^{n} \delta_i}{\sum_{i=1}^{n} T_i} \, .$$

For the piecewise exponential model, we can go through similar (but a bit more tedious) calculations to get k MLEs: for $j = 1, 2, \cdots, k$,

$$\hat{\lambda}_j = \frac{\sum_{i=1}^{n} \delta_i I[t_{j-1} \leq T_i < t_j]}{\sum_{i=1}^{n} (t_j - t_{j-1})I[T_i > t_j] + \sum_{i=1}^{n} (T_i - t_{j-1})I[t_{j-1} \leq T_i < t_j]} \, .$$

Although the formula looks a bit long, the interpretations are straightforward: the numerator is the number of observed failures within the interval $[t_{j-1}, t_j)$; the denominator is the total time spent in the interval $[t_{j-1}, t_j)$ by all subjects. This interpretation is also applicable to the estimator for the simple exponential model. We notice this estimator $\hat{\lambda}_j$ only involves what happens within the jth piece $[t_{j-1}, t_j)$, and does not depend on how many observations T_i, if any, are smaller than t_{j-1}, and also not on how long a patient survives after t_j.

Furthermore, taking the second derivative of the log likelihood, we see that the off-diagonal elements of the Fisher information matrix are all zero. This implies that the (asymptotic) correlations between $\hat{\lambda}_j$ and $\hat{\lambda}_l$, $j \neq l$, are all zero. The approximate variance of the MLE $\hat{\lambda}_j$ from the (observed) Fisher information matrix, is given by

$$\frac{(\hat{\lambda}_j)^2}{\sum_{i=1}^{n} \delta_i I[t_{j-1} \leq T_i < t_j]} \, . \tag{1.6}$$

Interestingly, when the number of pieces grows to infinity and the maximum length of pieces shrinks to zero, the piecewise exponential model becomes a nonparametric model. The estimators we just derived will become nonparametric estimators. We shall come back to this after we introduce the nonparametric estimator of Nelson–Aalen in Section 1.1.5.

1.1.5   The Nelson–Aalen and Kaplan–Meier Estimators

The Nelson–Aalen estimator is a nonparametric estimator of the cumulative hazard function based on n independent identically distributed (i.i.d.) right censored observations.

Given a random sample of right censored observations

$$(T_i, \delta_i) \ ; \quad i = 1, 2, \cdots, n$$

we define

$$N(t) = \sum_{i=1}^{n} I[T_i \leq t, \delta_i = 1] \quad \text{and} \quad R(t) = \sum_{i=1}^{n} I[T_i \geq t] \ .$$

The Nelson–Aalen estimator is defined as

$$\hat{\Lambda}_{NA}(t) = \sum_{s \leq t} \frac{dN(s)}{R(s)} \ . \tag{1.7}$$

We recall $dN(s) = N(s+) - N(s-)$ is the jump size of $N(t)$ at s. Notice the sum on the right is a finite sum, since $N(t)$ has at most n jumps. In other words, the Nelson–Aalen estimator is the sum of a series of jumps, and the size of the jump at s is the number of observed deaths over the number at risk at time s.

The Nelson–Aalen estimator and the Kaplan–Meier estimator are connected by the formula

$$1 - \hat{F}_{KM}(t) = \prod_{s \leq t}(1 - d\hat{\Lambda}_{NA}(s)) = \prod_{s \leq t}\left(1 - \frac{dN(s)}{R(s)}\right) \tag{1.8}$$

and

$$\hat{\Lambda}_{NA}(t) = \int_0^t \frac{d\hat{F}_{KM}(s)}{1 - \hat{F}_{KM}(s-)} \ . \tag{1.9}$$

We notice this is just the formula connecting cumulative hazard to distribution we discussed in Section 1.1.1 for the purely discrete case.

The above definition of the Kaplan–Meier estimator (also the Nelson–Aalen) works for t all the way up to the largest observation of T_i, but says nothing about the estimator for t after the largest observation. The term $dN(s)/R(s)$ after the largest T_i is $0/0$ and is interpreted as value 0. The monotonicity requirement for the Kaplan–Meier estimator will force $1 - \hat{F}_{KM}(s) = 0$ for s after the largest observation, provided the last term in (1.8) or (1.7) has $dN(s)/R(s) = 1$. This, in turn, determines the Nelson–Aalen via (1.9). If the last term has $dN(s)/R(s) < 1$, there is no unique definition for the Kaplan–Meier or Nelson–Aalen estimator. To make things definite, we often let $1 - \hat{F}_{KM}(t) = 0$ for t larger than the largest observed T_i.

For later reference, we note that the empirical likelihood of the Kaplan–Meier does not depend on how the Kaplan–Meier (or Nelson–Aalen) is defined *after* the largest observation T_i (next section).

For various properties of the Kaplan–Meier estimator and the Nelson–Aalen estimator, we refer readers to standard survival analysis textbooks. The properties in which we shall be most interested in this book are (1) that they are the distribution function and the cumulative hazard function that maximize the empirical likelihood function, which we will discuss in the next section; (2) the law of large numbers and central limit theorem for the Kaplan–Meier and Nelson–Aalen estimators, which will appear in Chapters 2 and 3.

Kaplan–Meier Survival Curve

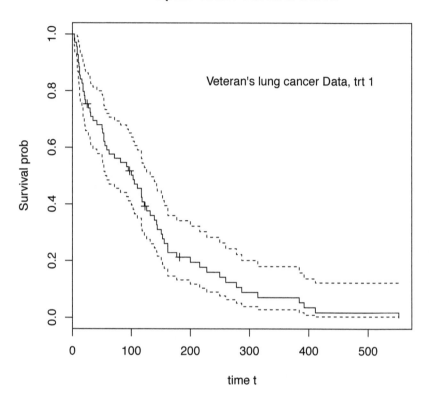

Figure 1.1: Plot of the Kaplan–Meier curve, with 95% pointwise confidence intervals by log transformation.

The Kaplan–Meier estimator is (sort of) unbiased; at least the bias is too small to worry about. It is also the "best" estimator of the survival probability when no parametric model is imposed. A very nice property of the Kaplan–Meier estimator is that it produces a plot of the estimated survival curve over time, which intuitively summarizes how the survival probability dwindles as time passes. Anybody could understand a Kaplan–Meier plot easily.

This plot is easy to produce in R thanks to the survival package. For a non-statistician, that may be the end of the story. But anyone with the slightest statistical sense will ask "how accurate is the Kaplan–Meier estimator?" Fortunately, there is a variance estimator for the Kaplan–Meier, the so-called Greenwood formula:

$$Var(\hat{F}_{KM}(t)) \approx [1 - \hat{F}_{KM}(t)]^2 \sum_{s \leq t} \frac{dN(s)}{R(s)[R(s) - dN(s)]} = \hat{\sigma}^2(t) . \qquad (1.10)$$

Unfortunately, the usual confidence interval (the so-called Wald confidence interval) does not work very well here. The reason: the survival probability is always between 0 and 1. So any sensible confidence interval should also be between 0 and 1. Another property of the survival curve is that the survival probability must decrease over time, and it is reasonable to expect the confidence intervals also have this monotone property. But the Wald confidence interval

$$1 - \hat{F}_{KM}(t) \pm Z_{\alpha/2} \sqrt{\hat{\sigma}^2(t)}$$

has neither of these two properties. (To be precise, Wald confidence intervals are not guaranteed to have this property for all cases.) A possible solution is to use the Wald confidence interval *after* a transformation of parameter, and after you get the confidence interval, transform it back. The problem with that is that there are literally infinitely many possible transformations and there is no clear cut choice of one over the other. On top of that, the best choice might depend on t, i.e., the best choice depends on in which time period you want a good confidence interval. The current survival software (SAS and R, etc.) all provide several possible transformations to chose from[1] and recommend one based on past examples and simulations. But different software may recommend different transformations, e.g., SAS default is log-log and R function survfit in the package survival defaults to log.

Thomas and Grunkemeier's [112] suggestion is a great idea: use the likelihood ratio test with the Kaplan–Meier estimator but do it nonparametrically. And invert the test to obtain the confidence interval. Since the Kaplan–Meier estimator is a non-parametric version of the MLE, a nonparametric version of the likelihood ratio test seems a logical next step. Using their suggestion, numerous studies were conducted; the confidence intervals obtained by inverting the nonparametric likelihood ratio test are always among the best, if not the best confidence intervals.

Owen realized the generality of this new method and was first to systematically study and apply the method to all areas of statistical problems. He also coined the term "empirical likelihood" and is the author of the first book on the subject [81].

It is not clear why SAS and the R survival package do not include the Thomas and Grunkemeier confidence interval. In my opinion, this should be the default choice of the confidence interval. There does exist an R package km.ci that computes the Thomas–Grunkemeier empirical likelihood interval for all time t. Our examples later in Chapters 2 and 3 will show how to use the emplik package to get a confidence interval of survival probability at a given time t_0 (and much more).

Example 4 (continued) *We now come back to the piecewise exponential model example. Since the Nelson–Aalen estimator is an estimator of the cumulative hazard function $\Lambda(\tau)$, we examine how to estimate this quantity under the piecewise exponential model.*

First, under the piecewise exponential model the cumulative hazard function can be written as (to make the notation simpler, suppose in the piecewise exponential

---

[1] SAS proc lifetest provides log, log-log, arcsine-square root, logit transform; R survival provides log and log-log transform.

model the partition is such that $t_{j-1} < \tau < t_j$)

$$\Lambda(\tau) = \sum_{i=1}^{j-1} \lambda_i(t_{i-1} - t_i) + \lambda_j(\tau - t_{j-1}) \, .$$

Because the MLE is invariant, we just need to plug in the MLE where parameters appear to obtain the MLE of the cumulative hazard, and thus the MLE of $\Lambda(\tau)$ is just

$$\hat{\Lambda}(\tau) = \sum_{i=1}^{j-1} \hat{\lambda}_i(t_{i-1} - t_i) + \hat{\lambda}_j(\tau - t_{j-1}) \, .$$

If we use the approximation

$$\hat{\lambda}_m(t_{m-1} - t_m) \approx \frac{N(t_m) - N(t_{m-1})}{R(t_{m-1})} \tag{1.11}$$

then the estimator based on the piecewise exponential model can be simplified to

$$\hat{\Lambda}(\tau) \approx \sum_{i=1}^{j} \frac{N(t_i) - N(t_{i-1})}{R(t_{i-1})} \, .$$

We point out this last form of the estimator is almost the same as the Nelson–Aalen estimator.

We notice that (1.11) will be exact if the partition of piecewise exponential distribution is such that the cut points include all the observed values of survival times (and also the τ).

Also, because $\hat{\lambda}_i$ and $\hat{\lambda}_j$ are uncorrelated, and each variance $Var(\hat{\lambda}_j)$ can be estimated by (1.6), we can easily compute an estimator of the variance of $\hat{\Lambda}(\tau)$. First, we have

$$Var(\hat{\Lambda}(\tau)) = \sum_{i=1}^{j-1} Var(\hat{\lambda}_i)(t_{i-1} - t_i)^2 + Var(\hat{\lambda}_j)(\tau - t_{j-1})^2 \, .$$

After plug-in an estimators for $Var(\hat{\lambda}_i)$ from (1.6) and simplifies, by using (1.11), to arrive at an estimator

$$\hat{Var}(\hat{\Lambda}(\tau)) = \sum_{i=1}^{j} \frac{N(t_i) - N(t_{i-1})}{R^2(t_{i-1})} \, .$$

Compare this to one of the variance estimators Andersen et al. [3] discussed (their (4.1.6)):

$$\sum_{s \leq \tau} \frac{dN(s)}{R^2(s)} \, . \tag{1.12}$$

We would like to point out that the above does not constitute a general theory, and there are cases where things do not work out as expected. To identify the nonparametric problems that a comparable likelihood theory applies to is a question beyond the scope of this book. We will just point out that the empirical likelihood is a nonparametric counterpart of the parametric likelihood ratio test.

1.2 Empirical Likelihood

Even though the name empirical likelihood first appeared in 1988, the method actually was proposed earlier, for analyzing censored data in the survival analysis setting. Thomas and Grunkemeier [112] proposed inverting a nonparametric version of the likelihood ratio test to obtain confidence intervals for the survival probability based on the Kaplan–Meier estimator, although they did not use the name *empirical likelihood*. Thanks to Owen's pioneering work, empirical likelihood has attracted a growing list of researchers. Increasingly broader applications have been found, and empirical likelihood has become a recognized statistical tool in the nonparametric toolbox. Today there is a vast literature on the empirical likelihood method and its applications can be found in many areas of statistical sciences. Unfortunately, empirical likelihood procedures are not readily available in commercial statistical software yet.

1.2.1 Likelihood Function

The parametric likelihood function is a key concept in any standard statistical curriculum. The theory and methods based on the likelihood function, i.e., the maximum likelihood estimator (MLE), likelihood ratio test, Fisher information number, etc., are the cornerstones of modern statistical science.

The maximum likelihood estimator is generally an excellent estimator when the model has a finite dimensional parameter and some smoothness property. However, when the parameter of interest is infinitely dimensional (nonparametric), the story is mixed.

The most familiar example of a nonparametric maximum likelihood estimator (NPMLE) is the empirical distribution function. Kiefer and Wolferwitz [53] extended the definition of the likelihood function to include the nonparametric case. Based on a sample of i.i.d. observations, $X_i, i = 1, 2, \cdots, n$, they took the CDF itself, $F(t)$, as the parameter and showed that the sample distribution function $\hat{F}_n(t)$, or the empirical distribution function

$$\hat{F}_n(t) = \frac{1}{n} \sum_{i=1}^{n} I[X_i \leq t],$$

is the nonparametric MLE of $F(t)$. It is well-known that $\hat{F}_n(t)$ is uniformly consistent and shares most of the good properties of a (parametric) MLE.

Not long afterwards, Kaplan and Meier [52] calculated the nonparametric MLE of $F(\cdot)$ in the right censored data case, and the estimator is also well behaved.

However, there are also examples of dramatic failure of the MLE in the case when the dimension of the parameter grows with sample size n or is outright infinitely dimensional.

The general theory of NPMLE and the associated (asymptotic) distribution theory and optimality property similar to those of parametric counterpart are difficult and much effort has been spent on this subject. We refer readers to the book by Bickel et al. [8] for known results. The paper by Stein [105] is also very inspiring to read.

Example 5 *(Neyman–Scott) Suppose random variables Y_{i1}, Y_{i2} for $i = 1, 2, \cdots, n$ are independent and normally distributed: $Y_{ij} \sim N(\mu_i, \sigma^2)$. Here σ^2 is the parameter of interest and μ_i are the nuisance parameters. It is easy to verify the MLE of σ^2 is*

$$\frac{1}{n} \sum_{i=1}^{n} \frac{1}{2} \sum_{j=1}^{2} (Y_{ij} - \bar{Y}_i)^2 .$$

Clearly, this MLE converges to $\sigma^2/2$ instead of the correct parameter σ^2 as $n \to \infty$. Hence the MLE is inconsistent here. We point out this model involves nuisance parameters (μ_i) with dimension increases to infinity as sample size increases.

This example shows that when there are growing numbers of nuisance parameters, the MLE can be disastrous. On the other hand, many nice properties of the empirical distribution $\hat{F}_n(t)$, as an estimator for $F(t)$, are well-known. Although they are usually not derived from a general theory of the NPMLE but are due to the explicit form of the NPMLE, we can investigate the property of $\hat{F}_n(t)$ directly.

From this point of view, *empirical likelihood ratio test* is the nonparametric counterpart of the parametric likelihood ratio test and the Wilks theorem.

1.2.2   Empirical Likelihood, Uncensored Sample

Suppose $X, X_1, X_2, \cdots, X_n$ is a sample of i.i.d. random vectors in R^k from a population distribution F_0, which is assumed unknown.

For any CDF F, define the empirical likelihood function based on the observations $X_1, X_2, \cdots, X_n$

$$EL(F) = EL(F, x_1, \cdots, x_n) = \prod_{i=1}^{n} P_F(X = x_i) = \prod_{i=1}^{n} p_i \qquad (1.13)$$

where we denote $p_i = P_F(X = x_i) = F(x_i) - F(x_i-)$.

Among all the CDFs, continuous or discrete, the empirical distribution $\hat{F}_n$ maximizes the empirical likelihood function $EL(F)$:

$$\hat{F}_n = \frac{1}{n} \sum_{i=1}^{n} M_{x_i}$$

where M_a is a point mass at a.

The maximum value of $EL(F)$ achieved is easily seen to be $\prod_{i=1}^{n} 1/n$, since for the empirical distribution $\hat{F}_n$, we have $P_{\hat{F}_n}(X = x_i) = 1/n$. See, for example, Theorem 2.1 of Owen [81] for a proof.

Definition: The empirical distribution $\hat{F}_n$ based on n i.i.d. observations is a probability measure that puts $1/n$ probability on each of the observed values X_i in the sample.

Please note here that we allow the observations to be a k-dimensional random vector. In our applications later, we shall use it for the two-dimensional random vector (T_i, δ_i). In a regression context, we also would use it for the $(p+2)$-dimensional vectors (X_i, T_i, δ_i).

Next, we formulate the hypothesis and then explain Owen's empirical likelihood theorem or the Wilks theorem. The Wilks theorem for the empirical likelihood is at the center of this development.

The hypotheses we are interested in are about a finite dimensional feature of the infinite dimensional parameter: the CDF $F(t)$. We suppose the finite dimensional feature of F is given by $E_F g(X) = \int g(t) dF(t)$, where $g(t)$ is a given $R^k \to R^p$ function.

When $k = 1, p = 1$, then we are dealing with random variables (not vectors) and a parameter that is the mean of $g(X)$. Examples in this situation are easier to understand. But we do allow $k > 1$ and/or $p > 1$.

Example 6 *Assume $k = 1, p = 1$. If $g(t) = t$, then this is the mean value of the $F(t)$. If $g(t) = I[t \leq a]$, then $E_F g(X) = F(a)$. For other choices of $g(t)$, the integration represents various other features of the infinitely dimensional CDF $F(t)$.*

Example 7 *Here $k = 2$ and the two-dimensional random vectors are (T_i, δ_i) for $i = 1, 2, \cdots, n$. The g functions are defined by*

$$g_j((T_i, \delta_i)) = \frac{h_j(T_i) \delta_i}{1 - G(T_i)}$$

for $j = 1, 2, \cdots, p$. This function was proposed by Koul et al. [62] in their study of accelerated failure time models. The G function in the above is the CDF of the censoring variable, and $h_j(t)$ is derived from the usual normal equations for regression models.

The hypothesis we shall be testing is

$$H_0 : \int g(t) dF(t) = \mu \quad vs. \quad H_a : \int g(t) dF(t) \neq \mu . \qquad (1.14)$$

The empirical likelihood ratio test is to reject the null hypothesis if

$$-2 \log \frac{\sup_{F \in H_0} EL(F)}{\prod_{i=1}^n 1/n} = -2 \log \sup_{F \in H_0} \prod_{i=1}^n n \, dF(X_i) \qquad (1.15)$$

is too large. In the above expression, the sup over F is taken for those CDF that satisfy the null hypothesis, i.e., those $F(t)$ that $E_F g(X) = \mu$.

Let $p_i = dF(X_i)$; then the above empirical likelihood ratio statistic can be written as

$$-2 \log \sup_{p_i} \prod_{i=1}^n p_i n ; \quad \text{where} \quad \sum p_i = 1, \ \sum p_i g(x_i) = \mu . \qquad (1.16)$$

Owen showed (by using the Lagrange multiplier) that the p_i that achieve the supremum above are given by

$$p_i = \frac{1}{n} \frac{1}{1 + \lambda^\top [g(x_i) - \mu]} \tag{1.17}$$

and $\lambda \in R^p$ is obtained from the equation

$$0 = \frac{1}{n} \sum_{i=1}^{n} \frac{g(x_i) - \mu}{1 + \lambda^\top [g(x_i) - \mu]} .$$

Next Owen proved the following theorem about the asymptotic null distribution of the empirical likelihood ratio test, which we can use to set the threshold value when deciding if we should reject the null hypothesis with a given type I error α.

Theorem 1 *(Owen) Suppose $X_1, \cdots, X_n$ is a random sample of i.i.d. observations with a CDF F_0. Assume the random vector $g(X_1) \in R^p$ has a finite and positive definite $(p \times p)$ variance-covariance matrix. Let $\mu_0 = \int g(t)dF_0(t)$. Then, under the null hypothesis $\mu = \mu_0$ (i.e., the hypothesis (1.14)), we have*

$$-2 \log \sup_{p_i} \prod_{i=1}^{n} n p_i \xrightarrow{\mathcal{D}} \chi_p^2$$

as $n \to \infty$. The supremum above is taken for $\sum p_i = 1, \sum g(x_i)p_i = \mu_0$.

In fact, Owen showed that, under the null and local alternative hypothesis $\mu = \mu_0 + C/\sqrt{n}$, where C is a constant, we have

$$-2 \log \sup_{p_i} \prod_{i=1}^{n} n p_i = n(\bar{g}(X) - \mu)^\top \Sigma^{-1} (\bar{g}(X) - \mu) + o_p(1)$$

where

$$\bar{g}(X) = \frac{1}{n} \sum_{i=1}^{n} g(X_i)$$

and Σ is a symmetric matrix with elements

$$\Sigma_{ij} = \frac{1}{n} \sum_{k=1}^{n} (g_i(x_k) - \bar{g}_i(X))(g_j(x_k) - \bar{g}_j(X)) .$$

In other words, Σ is $(n-1)/n$ times the sample variance-covariance matrix.

Another way to summarize the above is to say that the empirical likelihood ratio test is asymptotically equivalent to the Hotelling T^2 test at the null hypothesis and local alternative, and thus has the same power for these situations asymptotically.

The above results and proof can all be found in the book by Owen [81]. It even contains a triangular array version of the above EL theorem with $X_{n,j}$. We would like to make some simple observations: in the proof of the above results, all Owen needed was (1) the central limit theorem for $\sqrt{n}(\bar{X} - \mu_0)$; (2) the variance-covariance matrix of the above limiting normal distribution can be consistently estimated by a sample variance-covariance matrix; and (3) the weak law of large numbers for $\bar{X}$, plus some way of handling the remainder terms in a Taylor expansion which may involve the law of large numbers for a high moment of X.

These properties are often satisfied by a martingale difference sequence, provided some mild regularity conditions are imposed. In fact, we have the following theorem. Without loss of generality assume $\mu_0 = 0$ and $g(t) = t$. Let $Y_{n,j} = X_{n,j}/\sqrt{n}$.

Theorem 2 *(Schick) Let $\mathcal{F}_{n,0}, \cdots \mathcal{F}_{n,n}$ denote a filtration for each n. Suppose that $Y_{n,j}$ is a k-dimensional random vector measurable with respect to $\mathcal{F}_{n,j}$ and $E[Y_{n,j} \mid \mathcal{F}_{n,j-1}] = 0$, for $1 \le j \le n$. Then the empirical likelihood ratio Wilks Theorem (Theorem 1) also hold provided the following two conditions are satisfied.*
(i) $\sum_{j=1}^{n} E[Y_{n,j} Y_{n,j}^{\top} \mid \mathcal{F}_{n,j-1}] = A_k + o_P(1)$, where A_k is a $k \times k$ invertible matrix.
(ii) (conditional Lindeberg condition)

$$\sum_{j=1}^{n} E[\| Y_{n,j} \|^2 I[\| Y_{n,j} \| > \varepsilon] \mid \mathcal{F}_{n,j-1}] = o_P(1) \text{ for every } \varepsilon > 0 .$$

PROOF: See Schick [102] □

An easier to check sufficient condition for (ii) above is the conditional Lyapunov condition:

$$\sum_{j=1}^{n} E[\| Y_{n,j} \|^{\alpha} \mid \mathcal{F}_{n,j-1}] = o_P(1) \text{ for some } \alpha > 2 .$$

In later applications, we will apply this theorem to the counting process martingales arising from right censored data in the context of Cox models and accelerated failure time models.

1.3 Empirical Likelihood for Right Censored Data

Consider again the right censored survival data

$$3+, 6, 2.2, 8+, 12, \cdots.$$

They are commonly recorded in software as two vectors, instead of a plus, with $(T_1, \delta_1) = (3, 0)$, $(T_2, \delta_2) = (6, 1)$, etc.

Assume $(T_1, \delta_1), (T_2, \delta_2), \cdots$ are i.i.d. (two-dimensional) random vectors from a two-dimensional distribution, with one component continuous (T) and one component discrete (δ, with only two possible values).

The likelihood function is the probability of the observed sample under the assumed distribution function (either a parametric or nonparametric distribution):

$$\prod_{i=1}^{n} P(T = t_i, D = \delta_i) = \prod_{i=1}^{n} p_i . \tag{1.18}$$

Remark: Here p_i is the joint probability for the observed value (T_i, δ_i).

This somewhat awkward two-dimensional distribution $P(T = t, D = \delta)$ can equivalently be written as two one-dimensional sub-distributions or sub-survival functions

$$U_1(t) = P(T > t, \delta = 1) \quad \text{and} \quad U_0(t) = P(T > t, \delta = 0). \qquad (1.19)$$

By equivalent we mean a 1 to 1 correspondence, i.e., given the two-dimensional joint distribution $P(T = t, D = \delta)$, we can derive the two sub-survival functions U_1 and U_0. Conversely, given the two sub-survival functions U_1 and U_0, we can determine the joint distribution $P(T = t, D = \delta)$.

Using these two sub-survival functions, the likelihood can be written as

$$\prod_{i=1}^{n} \{-\Delta U_1(T_i)\}^{\delta_i} \{-\Delta U_0(T_i)\}^{1-\delta_i}.$$

Here $\Delta U_1(t) = U_1(t+) - U_1(t-) = -P(T = t, \delta = 1)$, etc.

Until now we only assumed i.i.d.-ness of the (T_i, δ_i) vectors, or patient to patient i.i.d. If we further assume the random independent censoring model (see Section 1.1.2), that is, the plus sign in the data is due to an independent follow-up time C_i being shorter than the associated lifetime X_i

$$T_i = \min(X_i, C_i) \quad \text{and} \quad \delta_i = I[X_i \leq C_i]$$

then we have

$$U_1(t) = P(T > t, \delta = 1) = \int_t^\infty 1 - G(s)dF(s) \qquad (1.20)$$

and

$$U_0(t) = P(T > t, \delta = 0) = \int_t^\infty 1 - F(s)dG(s) . \qquad (1.21)$$

In the above we used $G(\cdot)$ to denote the CDF of C_i and $F(\cdot)$ to denote the CDF of X_i.

It can be shown that the two sub-survival functions, U_0 and U_1, are also equivalent to the two proper distributions, $F(s)$ and $G(s)$, under the independent random censorship model.

Remark: (identifiability) If we do not assume independence, then there are many choices of F and G with various degrees of dependence, and all of them will give the same sub-survival functions U_1 and U_0. See Tsiatis [115].

Assuming independent censoring and given n i.i.d. observations, (T_i, δ_i), the likelihood function can further be written in terms of F and G:

$$\prod_{i=1}^{n} [(1 - G(t_i))dF(t_i)]^{\delta_i} [(1 - F(t_i))dG(t_i)]^{1-\delta_i} . \qquad (1.22)$$

In most cases, we are mainly concerned with the inference of $F(\cdot)$, not $G(\cdot)$, since G contains information related to the quality of follow-up time. Only F contains information about survival. So the terms that do not involve F are considered constants, and the likelihood (concerning F) is proportional to

$$\prod_{i=1}^{n} [dF(t_i)]^{\delta_i} [1 - F(t_i)]^{1-\delta_i} . \qquad (1.23)$$

The log likelihood is, up to a constant term,

$$\log EL_1 = \sum_{i=1}^{n} \delta_i \log dF(t_i) + (1 - \delta_i) \log[1 - F(t_i)] . \qquad (1.24)$$

If all the observations are completely observed, i.e., no censor (all $\delta = 1$), then the likelihood function is just

$$\prod_i dF(t_i) . \qquad (1.25)$$

This last likelihood is often written as

$$\prod p_i \quad \text{with} \quad \sum p_i \leq 1.$$

Remark: Notice the different meanings of p_i here and in (1.18), where p_i is for the two-dimensional joint probabilities.

When there are some censored observations, the maximization of (1.24) is obtained by a discrete distribution, the so-called Kaplan–Meier estimator [52].

Remark: If the observed data is merely independent but not identically distributed (as in a regression setting), then the final (log) likelihood is similar to (1.24) except that CDF $F(\cdot)$ will become $F_i(\cdot)$.

1.3.1 Likelihood Function in Terms of Hazard

Because cumulative hazard functions and cumulative distribution functions have 1 to 1 correspondence, this censored empirical likelihood can be written in terms of the hazard. However, due to the continuous/discrete version of the formula, we may end up with several versions of the likelihood.

Poisson version of the likelihood:

Let $\Lambda(t)$ denote the cumulative hazard function for the random variable X_i. By using the relation

$$1 - F(t) = e^{-\Lambda(t)}, \qquad (1.26)$$

the contribution to the log empirical likelihood for a single observation (T_i, δ_i) is

$$\delta_i \log dF(t_i) + (1 - \delta_i) \log[1 - F(t_i)] = \delta_i \log \Delta\Lambda(t_i) - \Lambda(t_i) . \qquad (1.27)$$

However, the CDF F that achieves the maximum of log likelihood, the Kaplan–Meier estimator, is discrete; thus the use of $1 - F(t) = e^{-\Lambda(t)}$ is questionable. If we assume a purely discrete Λ, then the function value of $\Lambda(t)$ at t is just the sum of all jumps that occur before and up to t. Therefore, the log likelihood contribution is

$$\delta_i \log \Delta\Lambda(t_i) - \sum_j \Delta\Lambda(t_j) I[t_j \leq t_i]. \qquad (1.28)$$

For the log likelihood based on n i.i.d. observations, it is just the sum of n terms, each similar to the above:

$$\log EL_2 = \sum_{i=1}^{n} \left(\delta_i \log \Delta\Lambda(t_i) - \sum_j \Delta\Lambda(t_j) I[t_j \leq t_i] \right). \qquad (1.29)$$

If we assume merely independent but not identical distribution for the observations, the log likelihood will be a sum with terms that has its own Λ_i.

Remark: By a simple calculation, we can verify that among all cumulative hazard functions, the one that maximizes $\log EL_2$ is none other than the Nelson–Aalen estimator, $\hat{\Lambda}_{NA}$, based on n observations.

Remark: The careful reader may detect some inconsistency: we used a formula (1.26) which only works for the continuous case when deriving (1.27) but later assumes a purely discrete Λ in going from (1.27) to (1.28).

If the underlying distribution for the survival times is continuous, and the cumulative hazard functions/distribution functions we work with all have jump sizes shrinking to zero as the sample size grows, then the inconsistency should diminish. But if the true survival distribution is discrete, then the discrepancy will stay even as the sample size grows to infinity.

Binomial version of the likelihood:

Here we always stick to the discrete version of the CDF/hazard function. By using the relation (that applies to the discrete CDF/hazard)

$$1 - F(t) = \prod_{s \leq t} [1 - \Delta\Lambda(s)]$$

the contribution to the log empirical likelihood for a single observation (T_i, δ_i) is

$$\delta_i \log \Delta\Lambda(t_i) + \sum_j I[t_j < t_i] \log[1 - \Delta\Lambda(t_j)] + (1 - \delta_i) \log[1 - \Delta\Lambda(t_i)] .$$

Notice the last term is always zero (assuming that the cumulative hazard function $\Lambda(\cdot)$ does not jump when $\delta = 0$); we may simplify the above to

$$\delta_i \log \Delta\Lambda(t_i) + \sum_j I[t_j < t_i] \log[1 - \Delta\Lambda(t_j)].$$

Then the likelihood for n i.i.d. observations (T_i, δ_i) is

$$\sum_{i=1}^n \delta_i \log \Delta\Lambda(t_i) + \sum_{i=1}^n \sum_j I[t_j < t_i] \log[1 - \Delta\Lambda(t_j)].$$

Switching the order of summation on the second term, we have

$$\sum_{i=1}^n \delta_i \log \Delta\Lambda(t_i) + \sum_{j=1}^n \log[1 - \Delta\Lambda(t_j)] \left(\sum_{i=1}^n I[t_j < t_i] \right) .$$

Finally, using a different subscript for the double summation above (use t_s for t_i and t_i for t_j), the log empirical likelihood for n observations is

$$\log EL_3 = \sum_{i=1}^n \delta_i \log \Delta\Lambda(t_i) + \sum_{i=1}^n \log[1 - \Delta\Lambda(t_i)] \left(\sum_{s=1}^n I[t_i < t_s] \right) . \qquad (1.30)$$

One interesting observation is that the maximizer for the hazard empirical likelihood, using either the Poisson or binomial version, is always the Nelson–Aalen estimator:

$$\Delta \Lambda^*(t_i) = \frac{\sum_j \delta_i I[t_j = t_i]}{\sum_j I[t_i \leq t_j]}. \tag{1.31}$$

This can be verified by taking the derivative and setting it equal to zero in the log likelihood expression.

However, the Poisson version is easier to work with when we impose Cox model type constraints.

When we use a parametric approach to analyze censored data, the CDF/hazard functions are usually continuous and thus we use likelihood (1.24) or (1.29). When we use a nonparametric approach, the maximizer is usually discrete and thus we use the likelihood (1.24), (1.30) or (1.29), depending on if we are modeling the hazard or mean.

We notice the following fact: (1) for any discrete CDF $F^*(t)$ and its corresponding cumulative hazard function $\Lambda^*(t)$, we have

$$\log EL_1(F^*) = \log EL_3(\Lambda^*).$$

(2) For discrete CDF $F^*(t)$ and $\Lambda^*(t)$, while assuming the size of the jumps of $F^*(t)$ are shrinking to zero (uniformly) as $n \to \infty$, the two log likelihoods $\log EL_2$ and $\log EL_3$ will become close.

1.4 Confidence Intervals Based on the EL Test

The very first use of empirical likelihood was to construct better confidence intervals by Thomas and Grunkemeier [112].

Indeed, confidence regions/intervals constructed by inverting the likelihood ratio tests have many unique advantages. These good properties are well-known for (parametric) likelihood ratio tests. Since the empirical likelihood ratio test is a nonparametric analogy of the parametric likelihood ratio test, it inherits all the nice properties from its parametric counterpart.

Additionally, some of these advantages become more prominent in nonparametric settings.

(1) The likelihood ratio test statistic does not involve the calculation of an information matrix or variance explicitly. This is important because the (nonparametric) estimators in survival analysis often have intractable variances.

(2) An empirical likelihood ratio based confidence interval *does not* need any transformations. It is "transformation invariant." It is as if it knows which transformation is the best, and has already applied it *implicitly, automatically.* To achieve better small/medium sample properties, confidence intervals based on other methods often have to be constructed with a transformation. For instance, working on the parameter of a correlation coefficient, we use Fisher's Z-transformation. However, some parameters in survival analysis do not have an apparent default choice of transformation, and it is not clear what type of transformation is preferred. Also, in the case of a confidence band, different transformations might be needed for different t.

(3) The resulting confidence intervals/regions from inverting empirical likelihood ratio tests are always within the natural domain of the parameters (range respecting). This can also be viewed as the benefit of the "implicit best transformation."

Examples of confidence intervals illustrating the above advantages are abundant. We will supply a few in later chapters.

1.5 Datasets

This book does not contain datasets in printed form. Rather, we will make use of existing datasets that are available electronically online. In my experience, unless the dataset is very small and simple, a printed dataset is rarely used. Data entry is burdensome and error prone. People prefer datasets in electronic form and online.

Datasets used to illustrate the calculations in this book can all be found in the four R packages: (1) `survival`, which is a recommended package usually included in every R installation by default; (2) `KMsurv`, which is a package that includes all the datasets used in the survival analysis book of Klein and Moeschberger [59]; (3) `emplik`, the main R package for the empirical likelihood method, which includes all the functions to calculate the empirical likelihood ratio in survival analysis and also contains one dataset; (4) `ELYP`, which contains functions related to the empirical likelihood analysis of the Cox regression model and other hazard regression models. These four R packages can all be found in the online repository CRAN.

Additional user defined datasets should be first read into R before they can be analyzed. For instructions on how to read data into R please see, for example, [93].

1.6 Historical Notes

The definitions of the Kaplan–Meier estimator, the Nelson–Aalen estimator and the Greenwood formula are all in common use and can be found in many survival analysis books, including [51], [59] and [111].

Thomas and Grunkemeier [112], Li [67] used the so-called binomial version of the censored data empirical likelihood. Murphy [74] discussed the Poisson version of censored data empirical likelihood.

Most of the empirical likelihood definition and results in this chapter can be found in Owen [81]. In particular, Theorem 1 is due to Owen.

A comprehensive review paper over the development and application of empirical likelihood method in econometrics is Kitamura [57].

Censored data nonparametric likelihood is discussed in [52]. Li et al. [68] review the empirical likelihood literature related to survival analysis.

The empirical likelihood Wilks theorem for the Martingale differences has also been considered by Chen and Cui [13]. However, they only considered a one-dimensional case. Our version is based on Schick [102], who used Peng and Schick [86] in the proof.

1.7 Exercises

Exercise 1.1 *Write an R function that will generate random variables that follow a piecewise exponential distribution, say with 3 pieces with given cut points $t_1 < t_2$ and 3 rates $\lambda_1, \lambda_2, \lambda_3$.*

Exercise 1.2 *Verify the MLEs obtained in Example 4 for the exponential and piecewise exponential distributions.*

Exercise 1.3 *Verify the observed Fisher information matrix for the piecewise exponential distribution is indeed given as in Example 4.*

Exercise 1.4 *Assume the variance of the Nelson–Aalen estimator can be consistently estimated by (1.12). Derive an estimator of the variance of the Kaplan–Meier estimator using the relation $1 - F(\tau) = \exp(-\Lambda(\tau))$. Compare your result to the Greenwood formula (1.10).*

Exercise 1.5 *Assume the Nelson–Aalen estimator has independent increments, with a variance that can be consistently estimated by (1.12). Find a covariance estimator between $\hat{F}(t)$ and $\hat{F}(s)$ $(0 < s < t < \infty)$ of a Kaplan–Meier estimator, using the relation $1 - F(\tau) = \exp(-\Lambda(\tau))$.*

Exercise 1.6 *Given a sample of right censored data: (T_i, δ_i), $i = 1, 2, \cdots, n$. Suppose $\hat{F}_n(t)$ is the Kaplan–Meier estimator computed from this sample. Next we replace δ_i by $1 - \delta_i$ and compute the Kaplan–Meier estimator based on $(T_i, 1 - \delta_i)$. Call this estimator $\hat{G}_n(t)$.*
Show that $(1 - \hat{F}_n(t))(1 - \hat{G}_n(t)) = R(t)/n$, where $R(t) = \sum_{i=1}^{n} I[T_i \geq t]$.

Exercise 1.7 *Given the two sub-survival functions U_1 and U_0, derive the distributions F and G under the independent random censorship model. [The converse is already given as in the two integrals (1.20) and (1.21): determine the two sub-survival functions, U_1 and U_0, in terms of F and G.]*

Chapter 2

Empirical Likelihood for Linear Functionals of Hazard

As we pointed out in Chapter 1, a trademark of survival analysis is the introduction of hazard parameters. Although it is equivalent to a CDF, many statistical analyses of survival data become easier when we use the hazard function as the parameter. Empirical likelihood is another testament to that fact.

The drawback of using hazard as the parameter is that for continuous and discrete random variables, the formula may look different. We shall study the hazard empirical likelihood for survival data in continuous and discrete cases separately.

2.1 Empirical Likelihood, Poisson Version

Suppose that $X_1, X_2, \cdots, X_n$ are i.i.d. nonnegative random variables denoting lifetimes with a *continuous* distribution function $F_0(t)$ and cumulative hazard function $\Lambda_0(t)$. Independent of the lifetimes, there are censoring times $C_1, C_2, \cdots, C_n$ which are i.i.d. with a distribution $G_0(t)$. Only the censored observations, (T_i, δ_i), are available to us:

$$T_i = \min(X_i, C_i) \quad \text{and} \quad \delta_i = I[X_i \le C_i] \quad \text{for } i = 1, 2, \cdots, n.$$

This is the random independent censorship model we discussed in Chapter 1.

For the empirical likelihood of the above censored observations, we use the Poisson extension of the empirical likelihood as discussed in Chapter 1. It is defined as

$$EL(\Lambda) = \prod_{i=1}^{n} [\Delta\Lambda(T_i))]^{\delta_i} \exp\{-\Lambda(T_i)\} \tag{2.1}$$

$$= \prod_{i=1}^{n} [\Delta\Lambda(T_i))]^{\delta_i} \exp\{-\sum_{j:T_j \le T_i} \Delta\Lambda(T_j)\} \tag{2.2}$$

where $\Delta\Lambda(t) = \Lambda(t+) - \Lambda(t-)$ is the jump of the cumulative hazard at t. The second line above assumes a purely discrete $\Lambda(\cdot)$ that has possible jumps only at the observed times. The reason for this simplification is that we are looking to maximize the empirical likelihood over all hazard functions, and obviously only those discrete hazard functions are possible candidates for the maximizer(s). A similar situation appeared in [78], where Owen worked with distribution functions and restricted attention to

23

those purely discrete distribution functions that only have jumps at observed sample values $F(t) \ll$ the empirical distribution. Li [67] also showed that the above simplification of the empirical likelihood is consistent with the nonparametric likelihood defined by Kiefer and Wolfowitz [53]. Therefore, we shall restrict our attention in the EL analysis to those discrete hazard functions that are dominated by the Nelson–Aalen estimator $\Lambda(t) \ll \hat{\Lambda}_{NA}(t)$.

Let $w_i = \Delta\Lambda(T_i)$ for $i = 1, 2, \cdots, n$, where we notice $w_n = \delta_n$ because the last jump of a discrete cumulative hazard function must be one. This is similar to the requirement that all the jumps of a discrete CDF must add up to one. When the largest observation is censored, the NPMLE of the hazard function is not uniquely defined for t beyond the largest observation. This is similar to how the Kaplan–Meier estimator is not uniquely defined beyond the largest observation when it is censored.

The empirical likelihood at this $\Lambda(t)$ can be written in term of the jumps

$$EL(\Lambda) = \prod_{i=1}^{n}[w_i]^{\delta_i}\exp\{-\sum_{j=1}^{n}w_jI[T_j \leq T_i]\},$$

and the log likelihood is

$$\log EL = \sum_{i=1}^{n}\left\{\delta_i\log w_i - \sum_{j=1}^{n}w_jI[T_j \leq T_i]\right\}. \tag{2.3}$$

If we maximize the log EL above with respect to w_i (without constraint), we easily see that $w_i = \delta_i/R_i$ will achieve the maximum, where $R_i = \sum_j I[T_j \geq T_i]$. This is the well-known Nelson–Aalen estimator $\Delta\hat{\Lambda}_{NA}(T_i) = \delta_i/R_i$. If we define $R(t) = \sum_k I[T_k \geq t]$, then $R_i = R(T_i)$.

The first step in our EL analysis is to find a (discrete) cumulative hazard function that maximizes the log $EL(\Lambda)$ under the constraints (2.4) or (2.5):

$$\int_0^\infty g_1(t)d\Lambda(t) = \theta_1$$

$$\int_0^\infty g_2(t)d\Lambda(t) = \theta_2 \tag{2.4}$$

$$\cdots \cdots$$

$$\int_0^\infty g_p(t)d\Lambda(t) = \theta_p$$

where $g_i(t)(i = 1, 2, \cdots, p)$ are given functions that satisfy some moment conditions (specified later), and θ_i $(i = 1, 2, \cdots, p)$ are given constants. The constraints (2.4) can be written as (for discrete hazard and in terms of w_i)

$$\sum_{i=1}^{n}g_1(T_i)w_i = \theta_1$$

$$\sum_{i=1}^{n}g_2(T_i)w_i = \theta_2 \tag{2.5}$$

$$\cdots \quad \cdots$$

$$\sum_{i=1}^{n} g_p(T_i) w_i = \theta_p .$$

For $k = 1, 2, \cdots, p$, when θ_k takes its true population values, i.e., when $\theta_k = \theta_{0k} = \int g_k(t) d\Lambda_0(t)$, we call (2.5) the null hypothesis. When θ_k is only $O(1/\sqrt{n})$ away from the true population values, we call this the local alternative hypothesis.

2.2   Feasibility of the Constraints (2.5)

Obviously, if $g_j(t)$ is positive and θ_j is negative, then the jth constraint of (2.5) is impossible or *not feasible*. We shall call the pair $(g_j(t), \theta_j)$ *feasible* if the equation $\int g_j(t) d\Lambda(t) = \theta_j$ has (at least one) solution and the corresponding $\Lambda(t)$ is truly a hazard function.

Recall the Nelson–Aalen estimator, $\hat{\Lambda}_{NA}(t)$, is the NPMLE of the cumulative hazard function, thus $\hat{\theta} = \int g(t) d\hat{\Lambda}_{NA}(t)$ is the NPMLE of the true θ value. For a given $g(t)$, the θ value $\hat{\theta}_{NPMLE} = \int g(t) d\hat{\Lambda}_{NA}(t)$ is obviously feasible since the Nelson–Aalen estimator is a solution (i.e., the NPMLE is feasible). Also, when the sample size grows, the feasible region of θ also grows. In other words, if you add more observations to the original sample, the feasible region of θ gets larger.

Pan and Zhou [84] explicitly calculated these feasible regions. But for our analysis of empirical likelihood tests and the related confidence intervals, we are mainly concerned with the θ values that are near the true value (i.e., under the null hypothesis or local alternatives). Since the NPMLE is consistent, in fact $|\hat{\theta}_{NPMLE} - \theta_0| = O_p(1/\sqrt{n})$, a θ value that is within $O_p(1/\sqrt{n})$ of the true value θ_0 is also within $O_p(1/\sqrt{n})$ of the NPMLE.

So when the sample size gets larger, the feasibility of the θ values within $O_p(1/\sqrt{n})$ of either the true θ_0 or within $O_p(1/\sqrt{n})$ of the NPMLE $\hat{\theta}_{NPMLE}$ will not be a problem. For smaller samples and for other uses of the empirical likelihood (for example, in the Bayesian analysis where we want to calculate the EL value for largest possible region of θ), the empirical likelihood value for the nonfeasible constraints may need to be carefully defined. We shall take the simple approach in this book of defining the log empirical likelihood ratio to be infinite if θ is not feasible.

No matter how one defines the empirical likelihood beyond the feasible region, one principle is obvious: the empirical likelihood achieves its maximum value at the NPMLE $\hat{\theta} = \int g(t) d\hat{\Lambda}_{NA}(t)$ and for any other θ values, the further it is away from the $\hat{\theta}_{NPMLE}$, the smaller will be the empirical likelihood value – a kind of monotone property.

We illustrate the feasible region using the dataset `azt` from the package `KMsurv`. There are 45 observations, with 25 right censored. We take the difference of `age` and `ageentry` as the observed survival times, which are both measured in months. In this example we take the $g(t)$ function as $g(t) = \max(0, (500 - t)/200)$.

This plot shows the θ values against the -2 log likelihood ratio values, $-2(\log lik(\theta) - \max \log lik)$, instead of the single likelihood $\log lik(\theta)$. Here the feasible region for θ is (approximately) $0 < \theta < 50$. So if you use a θ value outside

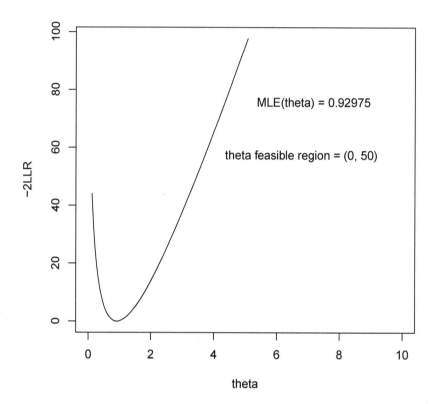

Figure 2.1: A plot illustrating the feasibility of theta.

this interval, the constraint (2.5) has no hazard solution. But as we can see from the plot, the most interesting places are when θ assumes a value near NPMLE = 0.92975. Since $P(\chi^2_{(1)} \geq 25) < 0.000001$, unless we are interested in the confidence intervals with a confidence level above 99.99999% or care about an exact p-value of a test smaller than 0.000001 (this is where the -2LLR values are larger than 25), those values of θ near the boundary are not really interesting.

In the subsequent analysis, we shall assume the constraints (2.5) are feasible, and there is no redundancy among the p constraints, i.e., these are genuine p *different* constraints.

We recall for the empirical likelihood setup considered by Owen, i.e., with i.i.d. data, no censoring and a mean constraint, all the feasible values of the parameter are precisely the convex hull of the observed data.

2.3 Maximizing the Hazard Empirical Likelihood

Since for discrete hazard functions, the last jump must be one, this implies that $w_n = \delta_n = \Delta\hat{\Lambda}_{NA}(T_n)$. The next theorem gives the other jumps of the hazard function under the constrain (2.5).

Theorem 3 *If the constraints (2.5) above are feasible (which means the constraint equations have a hazard solution), then the maximum of $\log EL(\Lambda)$ under the constraint (2.5) is obtained when*

$$w_i \quad = \quad \frac{\delta_i}{R_i + n\lambda^T G(T_i)\delta_i} \tag{2.6}$$

$$= \quad \frac{\delta_i}{R_i} \times \frac{1}{1 + \lambda^T(\delta_i G(T_i)/(R_i/n))} \tag{2.7}$$

$$= \quad \Delta\hat{\Lambda}_{NA}(T_i)\frac{1}{1 + \lambda^T Z_i} \tag{2.8}$$

for $i = 1, 2, \cdots, n$ where

$$G(T_i) = \{g_1(T_i), \cdots, g_p(T_i)\}^T, \quad Z_i = \frac{\delta_i G(T_i)}{R_i/n} = \{Z_{1i}, \cdots, Z_{pi}\}^T$$

and $\lambda = \{\lambda_1, \cdots, \lambda_p\}^T$ is the solution of the following equations

$$\sum_{i=1}^{n-1} \frac{1}{n} \frac{Z_{ki}}{1 + \lambda^T Z_i} + g_k(T_n)\delta_n = \theta_k \quad for \ k = 1, 2, \cdots, p. \tag{2.9}$$

PROOF: Use the Lagrange multiplier to find the constrained maximum of $\log$ EL. See [84] for detailed calculations. □

The main theorem of this chapter is the following Wilks theorem.

Theorem 4 *Let $(T_1, \delta_1), \cdots, (T_n, \delta_n)$ be n pairs of i.i.d. random variables representing right censored survival times as defined above in the independent censorship model. Suppose $g_i(t)$ $i = 1, 2, \cdots, p$ are given functions that satisfy*

$$\int \frac{|g_i(x)g_j(x)|}{(1 - F_0(x))(1 - G_0(x-))} d\Lambda_0(x) < \infty, \quad all \ 1 \le i, j \le p. \tag{2.10}$$

Furthermore, we assume the matrix Σ defined below is invertible. Then, $\theta_0 = \{\int g_1(t)d\Lambda_0(t), \cdots, \int g_p(t)d\Lambda_0(t)\}^T$ will be feasible with probability approaching one as $n \to \infty$ and

$$-2\log ELR(\theta_0) \xrightarrow{D} \chi^2_{(p)} \quad as \quad n \to \infty$$

where

$$\log ELR(\theta_0) \quad = \quad \max_{w_i} \log EL(\text{with constraints (2.5), and } \theta = \theta_0)$$

$$-\max_{w_i} \log EL(\text{no constraints})$$

$$= \log EL(w_i \text{ from (2.8), with } \theta = \theta_0)$$
$$- \log EL(\hat{\Lambda}_{NA}). \qquad (2.11)$$

We define the matrix A and Σ as

$$\Sigma = (\Sigma_{kr}) = \int \frac{g_k(x)g_r(x)}{(1 - F_0(x))(1 - G_0(x-))} d\Lambda_0(x) ; \qquad (2.12)$$

$$A = (A_{kr}) = \frac{1}{n} \sum_{i=1}^{n} Z_{ki} Z_{ri} .$$

We comment that the matrix Σ is the variance-covariance matrix of the asymptotic distribution of $\sqrt{n}[\hat{\theta}_{NPMLE} - \theta_0]$; see Lemma 6. Assuming this matrix to be invertible also guarantees there is no redundancy among the p constraints.

Before we proceed to the proof of the theorem, let us look at a few examples.

Example 8 *As an example, we test if the cumulative hazard at 3 years is equal to $\theta = -\log 0.4$ in terms of days and using the integration with respect to the g function, that is, $H_0 : \int I[t \le 1095.75]d\Lambda_0(t) = -\log 0.4$. This is equivalent to testing if the 3-year survival probability is equal to 0.6 (for continuous survival time).*

```
library(survival)
data(stanford2)
time <- stanford2$time
status <- stanford2$status
myfun <- function(t){as.numeric(t <= 3*365.25)}
emplikH1.test(x=time, d=status, theta=-log(0.4), fun=myfun)
```

The output shows −2LLR, which is the -2 log empirical likelihood ratio, of 0.8027874. This corresponds to a p-value of 0.3702613.

```
1 - pchisq(0.8027874, df=1)
## [1] 0.3702613
```

A 95% confidence interval for the cumulative hazard at 1095.75 days, $\Lambda_0(1095.75)$, can be obtained by inverting the test:

$$\{\theta \mid -2ELR(\text{test } \Lambda_0(1095.75) = \theta) < \chi_1^2(0.95)\} .$$

This task can be accomplished by trial and error on testing various values of θ. Or it can be done with the help of the findUL *function in the* emplik *package.*

```
myULfun <- function(theta, x, d){
        emplikH1.test(x=x, d=d, theta=theta,
        fun=function(t){as.numeric(t <= 1095.75)})}
findUL(fun=myULfun, MLE= -log(0.43), x=time, d=status)
## $Low
```

```
## [1] 0.6568022
##
## $Up
## [1] 1.029419
##
## $FstepL
## [1] 1e-10
##
## $FstepU
## [1] 1e-10
##
## $Lvalue
## [1] 3.84
##
## $Uvalue
## [1] 3.84
```

The output gives a 95% confidence interval [0.6568022, 1.029419]. The Lvalue *(*Uvalue*) is the value of the empirical likelihood ratio test reached at the lower (upper) end of the interval. For a 95% confidence level, this should be 3.84 (the 95th percentile from a chi squared distribution, df =1). This also offers an error check. Using the invariance property of the likelihood ratio confidence interval, we find that the 95% confidence interval for survival probability $P(X > 1095.75)$ is $[\exp(-1.029419), \exp(-0.6568022)]$.*

Next, we test the hypothesis that the median survival time is 2 years (2×365.25 days): $\int I[t \le 730.5]d\Lambda(t) = -\log 0.5$.

```
myfun1 <- function(t){as.numeric(t <= 730.5)}
emplikH1.test(x=time, d=status, theta=log(2),fun=myfun1)
```

One of the returned items from the R function is -2LLR, *which is the −2 log empirical likelihood ratio.*

```
## $'-2LLR'
## [1] 0.1231046
## ......
```

This gives a p-value of 0.7257 on a chi square distribution with 1 degree of freedom.

Now we proceed to the proof of Theorem 4. First, we need the law of large numbers and the central limit theorem for the Nelson–Aalen estimator and both can be proved, for example, via a counting processes technique. The following two lemmas are basically the law of large numbers and the central limit theorem for the quantities involved in the above two matrices A and Σ.

Lemma 5 *Under the assumptions of Theorem 4, we have, for $1 \leq k, r \leq p$,*

$$\frac{1}{n}\sum_{i=1}^{n} Z_{ki}Z_{ri} = \int \frac{g_k(t)g_r(t)}{R(t)/n}d\hat{\Lambda}_{NA}(t) \xrightarrow{P} \int \frac{g_k(x)g_r(x)}{(1-F_0(x))(1-G_0(x-))}d\Lambda_0(x)$$

as $n \to \infty$ where

$$R(t) = \sum_{i=1}^{n} I_{[T_i \geq t]}.$$

Lemma 6 *Under the assumptions of Theorem 4, we have*

$$\sqrt{n}(\frac{1}{n}\sum_{i=1}^{n} Z_i - \theta_0) = \sqrt{n}(\sum_{i=1}^{n} G(T_i)\Delta\hat{\Lambda}_{NA}(T_i) - \theta_0) \xrightarrow{D} N(0, \Sigma)$$

as $n \to \infty$ where the limiting variance-covariance matrix is

$$(\Sigma_{kr}) = \int \frac{g_k(x)g_r(x)}{(1-F_0(x))(1-G_0(x-))}d\Lambda_0(x) \quad \text{for } 1 \leq k, r \leq p; \tag{2.13}$$

and

$$\theta_0 = \{\int g_1(t)d\Lambda_0(t), \cdots, \int g_p(t)d\Lambda_0(t)\}^T.$$

The proofs of the two lemmas appear in the next section.

Since the matrix $A \to \Sigma$ as $n \to \infty$ (Lemma 5) and we assumed Σ is invertible and thus positive definite, we conclude that for large enough n the symmetric matrix A is also invertible.

Let us denote the solution of (2.9) as λ^*. Given that the solution λ^* is small in absolute value ($|\lambda^*| = O_p(1/\sqrt{n})$ verified in the next section), we can expand the equations (2.9). Using the expansion, we can show that the solution of λ^* to the constraint equations (2.9) satisfies

$$\lambda^* = A^{-1}b + o_p(n^{-1/2}) \tag{2.14}$$

where

$$b = \{\frac{1}{n}\sum_{i=1}^{n} Z_{1i} - \theta_1, \cdots, \frac{1}{n}\sum_{i=1}^{n} Z_{pi} - \theta_p\}^T.$$

Define

$$f(\lambda) = \log EL(w_i(\lambda)) = \sum_{i=1}^{n}\left(\delta_i \log w_i(\lambda) - \sum_j w_j(\lambda)I[T_j \leq T_i]\right)$$

and the test statistic $-2\log ELR(\theta_0)$ can be expressed as

$$\begin{aligned} -2\log ELR &= 2[f(0) - f(\lambda^*)] \\ &= 2[f(0) - f(0) - \lambda^{*T}f'(0) - 1/2\lambda^{*T}f''(0)\lambda^* + o_p(1)]. \end{aligned} \tag{2.15}$$

Straightforward calculations show $f'(0) = 0$ and $f''(0) = nA$. Therefore,

$$-2\log ELR = -\lambda^{*T} f''(0)\lambda^* + o_p(1). \tag{2.16}$$

Plug in the expression for λ^*, (2.14), and simplify it to

$$-2\log ELR(\theta_0) = nb^T A^{-1} b + o_p(1).$$

Finally, by Lemma 5 and Lemma 6, we get

$$-2\log ELR(\theta_0) \xrightarrow{D} \chi^2_{(p)} \quad as \quad n \to \infty.$$

This proves Theorem 4.

Remark: The conclusions of the above theorem still hold if we replace the null value θ_0 with a sequence $\theta_{n0} = \theta_0 + o(1/\sqrt{n})$. This can be easily proved by rechecking every step of the above proof. In particular, verify the two lemmas. The change of order $o_p(1/\sqrt{n})$ in θ_0 does not affect the leading term in the $-2\log ELR$ approximation we considered in Theorem 4.

This fact will be important in later chapters when we replace the null hypothesis with some other equations that are only $o(1/\sqrt{n})$ different from the null considered here.

2.4   Some Technical Details

We now give a proof of Lemma 5, the law of large numbers for Z_i or for the integral of Nelson–Aalen estimator. The result is obviously true if we impose more moment conditions. However, we try to give a proof that only assumes the finiteness of the limiting integration and without the extra moment condition. Also, we allow the $g(t)$ function to be a random sequence of functions. Notice here the random variables Z_i are not independent. Please note that in the following, we implicitly assume that $\max T_i$ is unbounded. If the support of T_i is bounded from above, some modifications of the proof are needed.

Lemma 7 (*Improved version of Lemma 5*) *Under the assumptions below, for given* $k = 1, 2, \cdots, p$ *we have*

$$\frac{1}{n}\sum_{i=1}^n Z_{ki}^2 = \int \frac{g_k^2(t)}{R(t)/n} d\hat{\Lambda}_{NA}(t) \xrightarrow{P} \int \frac{g_k^2(x)}{(1-F_0(x))(1-G_0(x-))} d\Lambda_0(x).$$

Assumptions (We omit the subscript k. These conditions should hold for all $k = 1, 2, \cdots, p$.):

(1) The limit must be finite, i.e., $\int_0^\infty \frac{g^2(x)}{(1-F_0(x))(1-G_0(x-))} d\Lambda_0(x) < \infty$;

(2) If we allow the weight function to be random, $g_n(t)$, then we need to assume that it converges uniformly in any finite intervals, i.e., for any $\tau < \infty$, $\sup_{t\le\tau}|g_n(t) - g(t)|$ goes to zero in probability and the ratio $\sup_i |g_n(T_i)/g(T_i)|$ is bounded in probability. These two conditions are satisfied by the empirical distributions, the Kaplan–Meier estimator and the Nelson–Aalen estimator.

Notice in the central limit theorem (CLT) of the martingales (Lemma 6) we will further require that $g_n(t)$ be predictable functions.

PROOF: We first show the law of large numbers for $\int_0^\tau *$ for any given finite τ:

$$\int_0^\tau \frac{g_n^2(t)}{R(t)/n} d\hat\Lambda(t) = \sum_i I[T_i \leq \tau] \frac{g_n^2(T_i)}{R(T_i)/n} \frac{\Delta N(T_i)}{R(T_i)} . \tag{2.17}$$

Subtract and add the term (recall $\Delta N(T_i) = \delta_i$)

$$\frac{1}{n} \sum_i I[T_i \leq \tau] \frac{g^2(T_i)}{[1 - H(T_i-)]^2} \delta_i$$

in the above and regroup; we get

$$(2.17) = \frac{1}{n} \sum_i I[T_i \leq \tau] \delta_i \left(\frac{g_n^2(T_i)}{[R(T_i)/n]^2} - \frac{g^2(T_i)}{[1 - H(T_i-)]^2} \right)$$

$$+ \frac{1}{n} \sum_i I[T_i \leq \tau] \frac{g^2(T_i)\delta_i}{[1 - H(T_i-)]^2} . \tag{2.18}$$

The first term above is bounded by

$$\frac{1}{n} \sum_i I[T_i \leq \tau] \left| \frac{g_n^2(T_i)}{[R(T_i)/n]^2} - \frac{g^2(T_i)}{[1 - H(T_i-)]^2} \right| \delta_i$$

$$\leq \sup_{t < \tau} \left| \frac{g_n^2(t)}{[R(t)/n]^2} - \frac{g^2(t)}{[1 - H(t-)]^2} \right| .$$

The term inside the absolute sign converges uniformly to zero, by assumption 2 on $g_n(t)$, and the well-known fact that $R(t)/n \to [1 - H(t-)]$ uniformly. Therefore, the reciprocal of it is at least uniformly convergent on $t \leq \tau$.

The last term in (2.18) above is an i.i.d. sum with respect to (T_i, δ_i). By the classic law of large numbers, it converges to its expectation, which is

$$E\left(I[T_i \leq \tau] \frac{g^2(T_i)\delta_i}{[1 - H(T_i-)]^2} \right) = \int_0^\tau \frac{g^2(t)}{1 - H(t-)} d\Lambda_0(t) .$$

By assumption 1 it is finite. This proves that the lemma holds for any finite τ.

We need to take care of the tail $\int_\tau^\infty *$. By assumption 1,

$$\int_\tau^\infty \frac{g^2(t)}{1 - H(t-)} d\Lambda_0(t)$$

can be made arbitrarily small by selecting a large τ (say smaller than ε/C).

Since the ratio $g_n(T_i)/g(T_i)$ and $[1 - H(T_i-)]/[R(T_i)/n]$ are both uniformly (in $\sup_{1 \leq i \leq n}$) bounded in probability (assumption 2 and the property of the empirical distribution function) we have that the term is bounded in probability by

$$\sum_i I[T_i \geq \tau] \frac{g_n^2(T_i)}{R(T_i)/n} \frac{\Delta N(T_i)}{R(T_i)} \leq C \frac{1}{n} \sum_i I[T_i \geq \tau] \frac{g^2(T_i)\delta_i}{[1 - H(T_i-)]^2} .$$

This summation/average converges to its mean (since it is an i.i.d. average),

$$C \int_\tau^\infty \frac{g^2(t)}{1 - H(t-)} d\Lambda_0(t) ,$$

the absolute value of which, in turn, is smaller than the pre-selected ε. This completes the proof. $\square$

The proof of Lemma 6 is a direct consequence of the martingale central limit theorem. See, for example, Kalbfleisch and Prentice [51] Chapter 5, Theorem 5.1 in particular.

Verification that $\lambda^* = \lambda_0$ is small.

We give a proof that validates the expansion of (2.9). In other words, we show the solution of (2.9) is small. We want to show $\lambda^\top Z_i$ is small uniformly over i. We shall denote the solution as $\lambda^* = \lambda_0$.

Lemma 8 *Suppose $M_n = o_p(n^{1/2})$. Then we have*

$$\lambda_n = O_p(n^{-1/2}) \quad \text{if and only if} \quad \frac{|\lambda_n|}{1 + |\lambda_n M_n|} = O_p(n^{-1/2}) .$$

PROOF: Homework. $\square$

Lemma 9 *If $X_1, \cdots, X_n$ are identically distributed, and $E(X_1)^2 < \infty$, then we have $M_n = \max_{1 \le i \le n} |X_i| = o_p(n^{1/2})$.*

PROOF: Since $\{M_n > a\} = \cup\{|X_i| > a\}$, we compute

$$P(M_n > n^{1/2}) = P(\bigcup_{i=1}^n (|X_i| > n^{1/2})) \le \sum_{i=1}^n P(|X_i| > n^{1/2}) .$$

By the identical distribution assumption, the above is

$$= nP(|X_1| > n^{1/2}) = nP(X_1^2 > n) .$$

Since $EX_1^2 < \infty$, the right-hand side above $\to 0$ as $n \to \infty$. A similar proof will show that, if $E|X_i|^p < \infty$, then $M_n = o_p(n^{1/p})$. $\square$

Lemma 10 *We compute*

$$E \frac{\delta_i g^2(T_i)}{[1 - F(T_i)]^2 [1 - G(T_i-)]^2} = \int \frac{g^2(t)}{[1 - F(t)][1 - G(t-)]} d\Lambda(t) .$$

Therefore, if we assume $\int \frac{g^2(t)}{[1-F(t)][1-G(t-)]} d\Lambda_0(t) < \infty$, then

$$M_n^* = \max_{1 \le i \le n} \frac{\delta_i |g(T_i)|}{[1 - F(T_i)][1 - G(T_i-)]} = o_p(n^{1/2}) .$$

PROOF: Use Lemma 9. □

Now, using a theorem of Zhou [134] which says the ratio

$$\max_{1 \leq i \leq n} \frac{R(T_i)/n}{[1 - F(T_i)][1 - G(T_i)]}$$

is bounded in probability, we can replace the denominator of M_n^* above by $R(T_i)/n$:

$$M_n = \max_{1 \leq i \leq n} |Z_i| = \max \frac{\delta_i |g(T_i)|}{R_i/n} \leq M_n^* \max_i \frac{[1 - F(T_i)][1 - G(T_i-)]}{R_i/n} = o_p(n^{1/2}) .$$

Now we proceed: denote the solution by λ_0. We notice that for all i, $1 + \lambda_0^T Z_i \geq 0$, since the solution w_i given in Theorem 1 must give rise to a legitimate jump of the hazard function, which must be ≥ 0. Clearly, $w_i \geq 0$ implies $1 + \lambda_0^T Z_i \geq 0$.

First we rewrite Equation (2.9) and notice that λ_0 is the solution of the following equation $0 = l(\eta)$.

$$0 = l(\lambda_0) = (\theta_0 - \frac{1}{n} \sum Z_i) + \frac{\lambda_0}{n} \sum_{i=1}^{n-1} \frac{Z_i^2}{1 + \lambda_0 Z_i} . \qquad (2.19)$$

Therefore,

$$\theta_0 - \frac{1}{n} \sum Z_i = -\frac{\lambda_0}{n} \sum_{i=1}^{n-1} \frac{Z_i^2}{1 + \lambda_0 Z_i} \qquad (2.20)$$

$$\left| \theta_0 - \frac{1}{n} \sum Z_i \right| = \frac{|\lambda_0|}{n} \left| \sum_{i=1}^{n-1} \frac{Z_i^2}{1 + \lambda_0 Z_i} \right| . \qquad (2.21)$$

Since for every term (at least when $\delta_i = 1$, or $Z_i^2 > 0$), we have $Z_i^2/(1 + \lambda_0 Z_i) \geq 0$. Therefore,

$$\left| \theta_0 - \frac{1}{n} \sum Z_i \right| = \frac{|\lambda_0|}{n} \sum \frac{Z_i^2}{|1 + \lambda_0 Z_i|} .$$

Replace the denominator $1 + \lambda_0 Z_i$ by its upper bound, then for any i we have

$$|1 + \lambda_0 Z_i| \leq 1 + |\lambda_0| M_n ,$$

we get a lower bound in the fraction

$$\left| \theta_0 - \frac{1}{n} \sum Z_i \right| \geq \frac{|\lambda_0|}{1 + |\lambda_0| M_n} \frac{1}{n} \sum_{i=1}^{n-1} Z_i^2 \geq 0 .$$

Since

$$\theta_0 - 1/n \sum Z_i = O_p(n^{-1/2}) \qquad (2.22)$$

(due to the CLT, Lemma 6), we see that

$$\frac{|\lambda_0|}{1 + |\lambda_0| M_n} \frac{1}{n} \sum Z_i^2 = O_p(n^{-1/2})$$

and obviously $\frac{1}{n}\sum Z_i^2 = O_p(1)$ (Lemma 5). Thus we must have

$$\frac{|\lambda_0|}{1+|\lambda_0|M_n} = O_p(n^{-1/2}) .$$

By Lemma 8 above we must finally have $\lambda_0 = O_p(n^{-1/2})$.

As a consequence, we also have $\lambda_0 M_n = o_p(1)$ and thus $\lambda_0 Z_i = o_p(1)$ uniformly for all i. $\square$

Remark: The conditions we have imposed in Theorem 4 are minimal. However, this theorem only addressed the first order asymptotic distribution under the null hypothesis. For the higher order results, more conditions are needed.

Similar calculations to those proving Theorem 4 but under a local alternative hypothesis, $\int g(t)d\Lambda_0(t) = \theta_n$, where $\theta_n = \theta_0 + O(1/\sqrt{n})$, will show that the asymptotic distribution of the empirical likelihood ratio becomes a non-central chi square distribution, similar to Owen's Theorem 2 [78].

2.4.1   The Constrained Hazard Under the Null Hypothesis

We examine in this section the distance between the constrained and un-constrained NPMLE of the cumulative hazard function. The constrained or tilted hazard is given in Theorem 3 with $\lambda = \lambda^*$. We denote this estimator by $\Lambda_{\lambda^*}(t)$. The unconstrained NPMLE is the Nelson–Aalen estimator. We notice that the Nelson–Aalen estimator is also equal to $\Lambda_{\lambda=0}(t)$. Therefore, the magnitude of λ^* is a kind of distance between the constrained and unconstrained hazard estimator, and we know $\lambda^* = O(1/\sqrt{n})$. On the other hand, the log empirical likelihood ratio *is* also a kind of distance measure between the two (infinitely dimensional) parameters $\hat{\Lambda}_{NA}(t)$ and $\Lambda_{\lambda^*}(t)$. However, we should look at a third measure of the distance: the sup distance between the two cumulative hazard functions here.

We claim that the sup difference of the Nelson–Aalen estimator to the tilted hazard estimator, $\Lambda_{\lambda^*}(t)$, is only $O(1/\sqrt{n})$ when the null hypothesis is true.

Lemma 11 *If the integration*

$$\int_0^\infty \frac{|g(t)|}{[1-F_0(t-)][1-G_0(t-)]} d\Lambda_0(t) \qquad (2.23)$$

is finite, then

$$\sup_{t\leq \max(T_i)} |\hat{\Lambda}_{NA}(t) - \Lambda_{\lambda^*}(t)| = O_p(1/\sqrt{n}) . \qquad (2.24)$$

If the above integration (2.23) is infinity, then we can only claim the convergence rate (2.24) in finite intervals:

$$\forall \tau \quad suppose \quad \int_0^\tau \frac{|g(t)|}{[1-F_0(t)][1-G_0(t-)]} d\Lambda_0(t) < \infty.$$

We have

$$\sup_{t\leq \min(\tau, \max(T_i))} |\hat{\Lambda}_{NA}(t) - \Lambda_{\lambda^*}(t)| = O_p(1/\sqrt{n}) .$$

PROOF: We only prove the first result; the second result follows similarly. From Theorem 3, we know the jumps of the $\Lambda_{\lambda^*}(t)$ are

$$\Delta\Lambda_{\lambda^*}(t_i) = \Delta\hat{\Lambda}_{NA}(t_i)\frac{1}{1+\lambda^*Z_i} \cdot$$

Therefore,

$$\Delta\hat{\Lambda}_{NA}(t_i) - \Delta\Lambda_{\lambda^*}(t_i) = \Delta\hat{\Lambda}_{NA}(t_i)\left[1 - \frac{1}{1+\lambda^*Z_i}\right]. \tag{2.25}$$

Recall $\lambda^* = O_p(1/\sqrt{n})$ and $\max \lambda^*Z_i = o_p(1)$ from the proof of the theorem. We have

$$\left[1 - \frac{1}{1+\lambda^*Z_i}\right] = \lambda^*Z_i + O_p([\lambda^*Z_i]^2) .$$

Therefore, the leading term of the difference (2.25) is, after summation over i,

$$\sum_i \lambda^*Z_i\Delta\hat{\Lambda}_{NA}(t_i) \le |\lambda^*|\sum_{i=1}^{n} |Z_i|\Delta\hat{\Lambda}_{NA}(t_i) .$$

The summation on the right-hand side converges in probability to the integral (2.23) by a similar argument as Lemma 7. Since the integral (2.23) is finite, the summation on the right is also bounded in probability. Finally, we know $|\lambda^*| = O_p(1/\sqrt{n})$; we see that the claim (2.24) is true. $\square$

Remark: The same conclusion of the lemma also holds under a local alternative, i.e., when θ is not the null value but only $O(1/\sqrt{n})$ away from the null value. The only place we used the null value θ_0 in the proof is in (2.22), and this obviously remains true if θ_0 is replaced by $\theta_0 + O_p(1/\sqrt{n})$.

This lemma says that in the analysis of the empirical likelihood ratio, we could restrict ourselves to those cumulative hazard functions that are dominated by the Nelson–Aalen estimator and (2) only differ from the Nelson–Aalen estimator by $O_p(1/\sqrt{n})$ in sup norm. This is true at least for asymptotic analysis and for analysis of the statistics under the null hypothesis and local alternatives.

The difference in the two corresponding survival functions is obviously also $O(1/\sqrt{n})$.

2.5   Predictable Weight Functions

So far in our discussion, the parameters we have dealt with are defined by $\int g(t)d\Lambda_0(t)$, with $g(t)$ being a fixed function. For certain applications (for example, log rank tests), we need to extend the result to allow the $g(t)$ functions to depend on sample size n $g(t) = g_n(t)$, and $g_n(t)$ may be random but predictable with respect to the filtration that makes the Nelson–Aalen estimator a martingale. These two changes do not alter the conclusions of Lemma 5 and Lemma 6, yet they extend the applicability of the empirical likelihood ratio test (Theorem 4).

Correspondingly, the null hypothesis will become, for $r = 1, \cdots, p$,

$$H_0 : \int g_{nr}(t)d\Lambda(t) = \theta_{nr}, \quad \text{where} \quad \theta_{nr} = \int g_{nr}(t)d\Lambda_0(t) \tag{2.26}$$

or

$$H_0 : \int g_{nr}(t)d[\Lambda(t) - \Lambda_0(t)] = 0 , \quad r = 1, 2, \cdots, p.$$

In other words, we are testing or comparing a one-dimensional feature of the infinite dimensional hazard function $\hat{\Lambda}_n(t)$ to $\Lambda_0(t)$, but this one-dimensional feature may change with sample size n and depend on the history up to but not including time t. Typical examples of such $g(\cdot)$ functions are those involving $1 - \hat{F}_{KM}(t-)$, $\hat{\Lambda}_{NA}(t-)$ and $1/n \sum_{i=1}^n I[T_i \geq t]$ and some simple combinations of those three functions.

Obviously, some conditions are needed to ensure the same Wilks theorem holds for the empirical likelihood testing procedure with the new weight function $g_n(t)$.

Theorem 12 *Consider the hypothesis (2.26). If the weight functions $g_{nr}(t)$ satisfy the following conditions, then the same Wilks theorem conclusion of Theorem 4 still holds.*

Conditions on $g_{nr}(t)$:
(1) The weight functions $g_{nr}(t)$ are predictable.
(2) As $n \to \infty$, $\sup_{t \leq \tau} |g_{nr}(t) - g_r^*(t)| \to 0$ in probability for any $0 < \tau < \infty$, where $g_r^*(t)$ are nonrandom functions that satisfy the conditions of Theorem 4.
(3) As $n \to \infty$, the following ratio is bounded in probability:

$$\sup_i \frac{g_{nr}(T_i)}{g_r^*(T_i)} .$$

We point out that $1 - \hat{F}_{KM}(t-)$, $\hat{\Lambda}_{NA}(t-)$ and $1/n \sum_i I[T_i \geq t]$ obviously all satisfy (1) and (2) above. As for (3), for the Kaplan–Meier estimator and the Nelson–Aalen estimator, the required result can be found in Zhou [135]. And finally, for $1/n \sum I[T_i \geq t]$ the boundedness of the ratio is a well-known result of the empirical process; see, for example, van Zuijlen [120].

2.5.1   One-Sample Log Rank Test

One cornerstone of survival analysis is the so-called log rank test. In most cases, it refers to a test comparing the survival times of two or more samples with right censored data. Although less common, the one-sample log rank test can be constructed similarly. It is a test comparing the survival times of a single sample to a standard reference population. The standard reference population is often constructed from a National Vital Statistics or US Census table. See Woolson [125] and Finkelstein et al. [27] for more details. Recently Sun et al. [110] suggested that for samples smaller than 50 the traditional one-sample log rank tests are conservative, and some corrections based on Edgeworth expansion were suggested. Wu [127], however, suggests some variation of the one-sample log rank test by modifying the variance estimator.

Here we use empirical likelihood to carry out the one-sample log rank test. Generally speaking, empirical likelihood procedures usually have very good small sample properties. Besides, no variance estimators are needed in order to calculate the EL test. Finally, further improvement may be achieved by replacing the chi square distribution with an appropriate t-distribution-square when determining the type I error.

Therefore, it seems worthwhile to conduct a large scale simulation, comparing the EL log rank test to the traditional normal approximation based test or its variations, like those suggested by Wu [127] or Sun et al. [110].

Suppose the standard population has a hazard function $\Lambda_0(t)$ and the Nelson–Aalen estimator based on the sample under test is $\hat{\Lambda}_{NA}(t)$; the one-sample log rank statistics are based on

$$\int_0^{\infty} R(s)d[\hat{\Lambda}_{NA}(s) - \Lambda_0(s)] \qquad (2.27)$$

where $R(t) = \sum_i I[T_i \geq t]$. Under the null hypothesis that the hazard of the population under test is no different from the reference population, the above log rank statistic should have zero mean.

Therefore, this one-sample log rank test can be cast into the testing problem we have considered by empirical likelihood:

$$H_0 : \int g_n(t)d[\Lambda(t) - \Lambda_0(t)] = 0 .$$

By allowing the weight function g to be random and predictable, the empirical likelihood theorem of the previous section will cover this one-sample test and a lot more useful cases.

Other weight functions, as long as they are predictable, to replace $R(t)$ are also possible and will result in other tests. For example, if the weight function becomes $R^2(t)$, we get the one sample Gehan test. Another possibility is to use $[1 - \hat{F}_{KM}(t-)]^{\alpha}$ as the weight function.

Example 9 *Taking the log rank test, i.e., $g_n(t) = R(t) = \sum_i I[T_i \geq t]$, we may rewrite the null hypothesis $\int R(t)d\Lambda(t) - \int R(t)d\Lambda_0(t) = 0$ as $\int R(t)d\Lambda(t) = \theta$ where $\theta = \int R(t)d\Lambda_0(t) = \sum_i \Lambda_0(T_i)$.*

We first take data from Woolson [125], who compared 26 psychiatric inpatients at University of Iowa hospitals to the reference population. The reference hazard is taken from an Iowa State mortality table (sex, age and admit year matched). According to his calculation, $\theta = \sum_i \Lambda_0(T_i) = 4.6331$.

```
library(emplik)
obs1 <- c(1,1,2,22,30,28,32,11,14,36,31,33,33,37,35,
                25,31,22,26,24,35,34,30,35,40,39)
status1 <- c(1,1,1,1,0,1,1,1,1,1,0,0,0,0,0,1,0,1,1,
                1,0,0,0,1,1,0)

temp11 <- Wdataclean3(z=obs1, d=rep(1, length(status1)))
temp12 <- DnR(x=temp11$value, d=temp11$dd, w=temp11$weight)
TIME <- temp12$times
RISK <- temp12$n.risk
fR1 <- approxfun(x=TIME, y=RISK, method="constant",
                                yright=0, rule=2, f=1)
theta <- 4.6331
```

```
emplikH1.test(x=obs1, d=status1, theta=theta, fun=fR1)
## $'-2LLR'
## [1] 14.60348
```

This value, 14.60348, is different from the usual log rank test. For example, Woolson obtained $(15 - 4.6331)^2/4.6331 = 23.1967$. *However, in a recent paper, Wu [127] advocated a modified log rank test and used simulations to show it is more accurate than the usual log rank test. Using his formula, we have* $(15 - 4.6331)^2/[(4.6331 + 15)/2] = 10.9481$. *Our log EL ratio statistic, with a value sandwiched in between the traditional and modified log rank tests, seems to echo the conclusion that "the traditional one-sample log rank test is conservative," but the EL modification is not as radical as Wu's modification.*

Now simulated data from exponential distribution, with exponential censoring. Suppose we are testing if the data comes from an exponential distribution with hazard 0.2 and cumulative hazard $0.2t$.

```
surT2 <- rexp(35, rate = 0.2)
cen2 <- rexp(35, rate = 0.1)
obs2 <- pmin(surT2, cen2)
status2 <- as.numeric(cen2 >= surT2)

temp21 <- Wdataclean3(z=obs2, d=rep(1, 35))
temp22 <- DnR(x=temp21$value, d=temp21$dd, w=temp21$weight)
TIME <- temp22$times
RISK <- temp22$n.risk
fR1 <- approxfun(x=TIME, y=RISK, method="constant",
                              yright=0, rule=2, f=1)

theta <- sum(0.2*obs2)
emplikH1.test(x=obs2, d=status2, theta=theta, fun=fR1)
```

2.6 Two-Sample Tests

The two-sample log rank test is much more common than the one-sample test we discussed above.

We assume, in addition to the observations (T_i, δ_i), $i = 1, 2, \cdots, n$, there is also available a second sample with randomly right censored observations (U_j, d_j), $j = 1, 2, \cdots, m$. The cumulative hazard function of the survival times from sample one is $\Lambda_1(t)$ and, for sample two, $\Lambda_2(t)$.

The theory for the empirical likelihood developed in the previous two sections can be readily extended to the two sample case to cover the two sample log rank test, where the null hypothesis is

$$H_0: \int g_n(t)d[\Lambda_1(t) - \Lambda_2(t)] = 0 .$$

Or, more generally,

$$H_0 : \int g_1(t)d\Lambda_1(t) - \int g_2(t)d\Lambda_2(t) = \theta .$$

The $g(\cdot)$ function that leads to the two sample log rank test is given by

$$g_1(t) = g_2(t) = g_{LR}(t) = \sqrt{\frac{n+m}{nm} \frac{R_1(t)R_2(t)}{R_1(t)+R_2(t)}} ,$$

where $R_1(t) = \sum_{i=1}^{n} I[T_i \geq t]$ and $R_2(t) = \sum_{j=1}^{m} I[U_j \geq t]$ are the number of subjects at risk from sample one and two at time t, respectively.

Since we assume the two samples are independent, the log empirical likelihood of both samples will be simply the sum of the two one-sample log empirical likelihoods.

$$\log EL = \sum_{i=1}^{n} \left\{ \delta_i \log w_i^{(1)} - \sum_{j=1}^{n} w_j^{(1)} I[T_j \leq T_i] \right\} \tag{2.28}$$
$$+ \sum_{j=1}^{m} \left\{ d_j \log w_j^{(2)} - \sum_{k=1}^{m} w_k^{(2)} I[U_k \leq U_j] \right\} .$$

Obviously the maximum of the above log empirical likelihood is achieved when $\Lambda_1(t)$ (respectively $\Lambda_2(t)$) is equal to the Nelson–Aalen estimator from sample one (two), or $w_i^{(1)}$ equal to the jumps of $\hat{\Lambda}_{NA}^{(1)}$, $w_j^{(2)}$ equal to the jumps of $\hat{\Lambda}_{NA}^{(2)}$. Let us denote the maximum value achieved as $\log EL(\hat{\Lambda}_{NA}^{(1)}, \hat{\Lambda}_{NA}^{(2)})$.

When maximizing the two-sample log empirical likelihood (2.28) under the constraint specified in H_0, it is not hard to show by the Lagrange multiplier that the jumps of the two cumulative hazard functions take the form

$$w_i^{(1)} = \frac{\delta_i}{R_1(t_i) + \lambda g_1(t_i)} \quad i = 1, 2, \cdots, n \tag{2.29}$$

$$w_j^{(2)} = \frac{d_j}{R_2(u_j) - \lambda g_2(u_j)} \quad j = 1, 2, \cdots, m \tag{2.30}$$

and the λ above is the solution of the equation

$$\sum_{i=1}^{n} \frac{\delta_i g_1(t_i)}{R_1(t_i) + \lambda g_1(t_i)} - \sum_{j=1}^{m} \frac{d_j g_2(u_j)}{R_2(u_j) - \lambda g_2(u_j)} = \theta .$$

Similar to the one-sample case, we have the following Wilks theorem.

Theorem 13 *Assume the null hypothesis holds, i.e., $0 = \int g_{LR}(t)d\Lambda_1(t) - \int g_{LR}(t)d\Lambda_2(t)$. As $n \to \infty$, assume $m/n \to c$ where $0 < c < \infty$; we have*

$$-2\{\log EL(\text{with } w_i^{(1)}, w_j^{(2)} \text{ from (2.29)}) - \log EL(\hat{\Lambda}_{NA}^{(1)}, \hat{\Lambda}_{NA}^{(2)})\} \longrightarrow \chi_{(1)}^2$$

in distribution provided the following is finite and positive:

$$\int \frac{P(T_i \geq t)P^2(U_j \geq t)d\Lambda_1(t)}{[(1-c)P(T_i \geq t) + cP(U_j \geq t)]^2} + \int \frac{P(U_j \geq t)P^2(T_i \geq t)d\Lambda_2(t)}{[(1-c)P(T_i \geq t) + cP(U_j \geq t)]^2}.$$

If the weight function $g_n(t)$ in the null hypothesis is of p dimension, then the degree of freedom for the chi square limiting distribution is p.

The last condition of the theorem merely says the asymptotic variance of $\int g_{LR}(t)d\hat{\Lambda}_{NA}(t)$ is finite.

Example 10 *We first implement a two-sample log rank test by using EL. We use the* `smallcell` *lung cancer data included in the* `emplik` *package. There are two treatments and a total of 121 cases.*

```
library(emplik)
data(smallcell)
x1 <- smallcell[1:62, 3]
x2 <- smallcell[63:121, 3]
d1 <- smallcell[1:62, 4]
d2 <- smallcell[63:121, 4]

temp11 <- Wdataclean3(z=x1, d=rep(1, length(d1)))
temp12 <- DnR(x=temp11$value, d=temp11$dd, w=temp11$weight)
TIME1 <- temp12$times
RISK1 <- temp12$n.risk
fR1 <- approxfun(x=TIME1, y=RISK1, method="constant",
                             yright=0, rule=2, f=1)

temp21 <- Wdataclean3(z=x2, d=rep(1, length(d2)))
temp22 <- DnR(x=temp21$value, d=temp21$dd, w=temp21$weight)
TIME2 <- temp22$times
RISK2 <- temp22$n.risk
fR2 <- approxfun(x=TIME2, y=RISK2, method="constant",
                             yright=0, rule=2, f=1)

flogrank <- function(t){fR1(t)*fR2(t)/(fR1(t)+fR2(t))}
emplikHs.test2(x1=x1, d1=d1, x2=x2, d2=d2,
               theta=0, fun1=flogrank, fun2=flogrank)
## $'-2LLR'
## [1] 7.247221
## ......
```

This leads to a p-value of 0.007101083 by chi square distribution with one degree of freedom. Compared to the `survdiff( )` *function of the* `survival` *package, the p-value for the same data is 0.008015535.*

The log rank test is designed for "proportional hazards" type alternatives and can have very low or no power at all if the alternative is "cross hazards." To make things worse, the cross hazards situation is hard to detect unless we have large sample sizes. Plotting the two Kaplan–Meier curves may or may not help, since a cross hazards alternative (which is different from cross cumulative hazards) does not necessarily lead to cross survivals. When both hazards and survivals cross, they cross at different locations. Typically, the survivals cross much later, where either the study had already been stopped or large variances for the Kaplan–Meier estimators make the plot untrustworthy.

One possibility is to use a test that combines the log rank test with another that is designed for cross hazards.

```
NN <- length(x1) + length(x2)
myfun7 <- function(t) {as.numeric((fR1(t)+fR2(t)) > NN*0.6)}
fWlogrank <- function(t) {myfun7(t)*flogrank(t)}
fBOTH <- function(t) {cbind(flogrank(t), fWlogrank(t))}
emplikHs.test2(x1=x1, d1=d1, x2=x2, d2=d2,
                    theta=c(0,0), fun1=fBOTH, fun2=fBOTH)
## $'-2LLR'
## [1] 19.29306
## ...
1-pchisq(19.29306, df=2)
## [1] 6.464951e-05
```

Notice we have used a chi square distribution with 2 degrees of freedom to calculate the *p*-value, since there are two constraints in the EL.

In many examples and simulations, this combined test has a slightly lower power compared to the log rank test when we deal with the proportional hazards alternatives, but have much higher power than the log rank test when the alternative is the cross hazards type. Please see Bathke et al. [6] for more details.

2.7   Hazard Estimating Equations

Qin and Lawless [92] discussed the use of empirical likelihood with estimating equations. Of particular interest is the case where the number of equations exceeds the number of parameters, the so-called over determined case. One of the results Qin and Lawless obtained is that the maximum empirical likelihood estimator under the over determined estimating equations is consistent and asymptotically normal and automatically becomes the best estimator, in the sense that the (asymptotic) variance is the smallest compared to the usual estimator derived from estimating equations. In particular, it is better than the so-called generalized method of moment estimator (GMM).

Similar to the estimating equations setting of Qin and Lawless, we study here the estimating equations that are defined through cumulative hazard functions and based on right censored data. In particular, we show that the maximum empirical likelihood estimator behaves similarly to the case Qin and Lawless studied, and the empirical likelihood ratio test has a chi square distribution under the null hypothesis.

The estimating equation in terms of hazard is not commonly used, but in survival analysis the use of the hazard to construct estimating equations makes analysis easier, as we shall see in the case study later. Also, in view of a general result later (Section 3.4), we may always *approximate* and *replace* the estimating equations formulated in terms of the CDF (3.5) (i.e., with the Kaplan–Meier estimator), by its relative with hazard, i.e., (2.37). Thus the theory we have developed, including the Wilks theorem, etc., for the hazard estimating equations, is readily translated into results involving estimating equations of the CDF.

Before we delve into the development of the empirical likelihood for the hazard estimating equations, we shall review the rank estimating equations for accelerated failure time (AFT) models. This is also a motivating example to study estimating equations for censored data.

2.7.1   The Semi-Parametric AFT model

The semi-parametric AFT model is basically a linear regression model where the responses are the logarithm of the survival times and the error term distribution is unspecified. It provides a useful alternative model to the popular Cox proportional hazards regression model for analyzing censored survival data.

Consider the linear regression model

$$\log X_i = \beta_0^\top Z_i + \varepsilon_i \quad i = 1, 2, \cdots, n \tag{2.31}$$

where Z_i is a p dimensional covariate and ε_i are i.i.d., with an unspecified distribution $F_0(t)$. Since we are only going to use the ranks in the estimation, the mean of ε_i is not identifiable. Another way to put it is to think that the intercept term of the regression model is absorbed into the ε_i. The parameter β_0 is a p dimensional vector to be estimated.

Due to censoring, we are unable to observe all the $\log X_i$'s. Let C_i be the censoring times for X_i. Assume C_i and X_i are independent given Z_i. The data we can actually observe consist of (T_i, δ_i, Z_i), where

$$T_i = \min(\log X_i, \log C_i) \; ; \quad \delta_i = I[\log X_i \le \log C_i] \; .$$

Starting with Prentice [88], many researchers have studied the rank-based estimation method in the AFT model with censored data, including Tsiatis [117], Wei et al. [124], Ritov [97], Fygenson and Ritov [30], Lai and Ying [64] and Ying [130]. A nice summary can be found in Chapter 7 of Kalbfleisch and Prentice [51]. Our notation will be similar to that used by Jin et al. [47].

Basically, the estimation method will first calculate the *residuals* $(T_i - b^\top Z_i, \delta_i)$, and then test if the residuals are i.i.d. or uncorrelated with the covariates. The estimator of β_0 is the b value that makes the test statistic the least significant.

For any given p dimensional vector b, define the (censored) residuals $(e_i(b), \delta_i)$ as

$$e_i(b) = T_i - b^\top Z_i \; , \quad \delta_i = I[\log X_i \le \log C_i] \; . \tag{2.32}$$

The rank estimator of the regression parameter β_0 is the root of the equations:

$$0 = \sum_{i=1}^{n} \phi(e_i(b))[Z_i - \bar{Z}(b, e_i(b))]\delta_i \qquad (2.33)$$

where $\bar{Z}(b, e_i(b))$ is the average of those covariates, Z_j, that the corresponding $e_j(b)$ is still at risk at time $e_i(b)$, i.e., $e_j(b) \geq e_i(b)$:

$$\bar{Z}(b, e_i(b)) = \frac{\sum_{j=1}^{n} Z_j I[e_j(b) \geq e_i(b)]}{\sum_{j=1}^{n} I[e_j(b) \geq e_i(b)]}. \qquad (2.34)$$

The function $\phi(\cdot)$ is a weight function, and different choices are available. If $\phi(\cdot) \equiv 1$, then the test corresponds to the log rank test and thus we call the root of the equation the "log rank" estimator of β. The weight $\phi(t) = R(t) = \sum_j I[e_j(b) \geq t]$ corresponds to the Gehan test, and the root of the equation will be called the Gehan estimator.

Depending on the distribution of the error term ε, other choices of the weight may increase the efficiency of the resulting estimator or make the computation easier.

We notice (2.33) is a set of p equations where $p = dim(\beta_0)$.

A large sample study of the rank-based estimator for the censored data AFT model is given by Lai and Ying [64], Ying [130] and several subsequent papers including Jin et al. [47], which also includes the treatment of the general weighting functions.

It is known that the rank-based estimator is consistent and asymptotically normally distributed, but the asymptotic variance expression of the rank regression estimator involves the derivative of the hazard function for the error term ε, whose distribution is assumed unknown. We recall that empirical likelihood ratio tests do not need to calculate variance explicitly, which is a blessing here.

We notice that the estimating equation of the rank regression can be written as

$$0 = \sum_{i=1}^{n} R(e_i(b))\phi(e_i(b))[Z_i - \bar{Z}(b, e_i(b))]\frac{\delta_i}{R(e_i(b))} \qquad (2.35)$$

where $R(t) = \sum_j I[e_j(b) \geq t]$. Recall the jumps of the Nelson–Aalen estimator $\Delta\hat{\Lambda}_{NA}(t_i) = \delta_i/R(t_i)$. If we replace $\delta_i/R(e_i(b)) = w_i$ and $e_i(b) = t_i$ in Equation (2.35), we have

$$0 = \sum_{i=1}^{n} R(t_i)\phi(t_i)[Z_i - \bar{Z}(b, t_i)]w_i, \qquad (2.36)$$

which is precisely the form of the hazard constraints we studied in Sections 2.1 and 2.5, except here the time is in the residual scale, and the parameter is denoted as β instead of θ.

Some quick checks will verify that $R(t)$, $\bar{Z}(t)$ are predictable functions in the residual time scale. Therefore, if our choice of the weight function ϕ is also predictable, an application of Theorem 12 will give us the following theorem.

Theorem 14 *Under mild regularity conditions the Wilks theorem holds for the empirical likelihood ratio for testing the hypothesis $H_0 : \beta = \beta_0$ vs. $H_A : \beta \neq \beta_0$, i.e.,*

$$-2\log ELR(\beta_0) \xrightarrow{\mathcal{D}} \chi_p^2 \quad as \ n \to \infty$$

when the null hypothesis is true.

Example 11 *We use the myeloma data to illustrate the empirical likelihood analysis for the rank-based estimator in the AFT model. The dataset includes 65 subjects and 11 variables. Among the 65 survival times, 17 are right censored. This data is available in the R package* `emplik`.

We shall fit an AFT model

$$\log(time) = \beta \log(BUN) + \varepsilon \ ,$$

where the data from `emplik` *provides the variables time and* $\log(BUN)$ *(blood urea nitrogen). So we need only to take a natural log of the time as the response for the AFT model.*

The empirical likelihood ratio test of the slope $\beta = -2$ *is obtained as*

```
library(emplik)
data(myeloma)
RankRegTestH(y=log(myeloma[,1]), d=myeloma[,2],
                    x=myeloma[,3], beta=-2)
RankRegTestH(y=log(myeloma[,1]), d=myeloma[,2],
             x=myeloma[,3], beta=-2, type="Logrank")
```

The default test is the Gehan test.

Table 2.1 summarizes the results of the empirical likelihood test. The confidence intervals can be obtained by testing a range of trial values of β *and then finding the tipping point for the 90% significance based on the -2 log likelihood ratio value. For more details, see Chapter 6 on the computing of empirical likelihood ratio and inverting tests to get confidence intervals.*

Table 2.1: Rank Estimators and Empirical Likelihood 90% Confidence Intervals for AFT Model β with the Myeloma Data

Weighting Function	Estimator	90% Confidence Interval
Gehan	-1.690	$[-2.466, -0.719]$
Log rank	-1.679	$[-2.623, -0.523]$

2.7.2 Overdetermined Equations

The hazard estimating equations we derived from AFT rank estimation in the previous section are in the form

$$\sum_{i=1}^{n} g_k(t_i,\beta)\delta_i w_i = 0; \quad k=1,2,\cdots,p, \tag{2.37}$$

where w_i is the jump of a cumulative hazard function. When w_i happens to be the jumps of the Nelson–Aalen estimator, the solution to these equations is our estimator $\hat{\beta}$. There is one and only one solution since there are p equations (in either Gehan or log rank) and the dimension of β is also p.

However, sometimes there are valid arguments to chose either one of two different weight functions in the rank estimating functions. For example, the Gehan weight will result in a monotone estimating function and thus make the root seeking algorithm robust [30], but a log rank weight (or the adaptive weight studied by Jin et al. [47]) may increase the efficiency of the resulting estimator in some situations. Unfortunately, the log rank weight destroys the monotone property and makes solving equations difficult. The empirical likelihood approach to the estimating equations provides another choice: that is, we may use *both* sets of equations together, hoping to reap the benefits of both.

This leads to the *overdetermined* estimating equations. Suppose we have r $(r>p)$ estimating equations in terms of the hazard

$$\sum_{i=1}^{n} g_k(t_i,\beta)\delta_i w_i = \mu_k; \quad k=1,2,\cdots,r, \tag{2.38}$$

where μ_k are given constants and β is a parameter of dimension $p<r$. These equations do not usually have a solution β when w_i are taken to be the jumps of the Nelson–Aalen estimator, since the number of equations (r) exceeds the number of parameters (p). However, for all β values near the true value, if r is small compared to the sample size n, and the r equations are "compatible," we can find a cumulative hazard function (tilted away from the Nelson–Aalen estimator) such that its w_i will satisfy all r equations. Intuitively, there are r equations and we have about n jumps of hazard w_i to work with. Therefore, we can expect some set of w_i that satisfy these r equations. However, we are looking for the solution in w_i that has the largest empirical likelihood value.

The maximum empirical likelihood estimator $\hat{\beta}$ is defined as the value β such that we need the least amount of tilting of cumulative hazard in order to satisfy all the r equations. The amount of tilting or the distance of tilting is measured in terms of the log empirical likelihood value. The smaller the empirical likelihood value of the hazard, the farther away it is deemed from the Nelson–Aalen estimator.

For given β, μ_k and functions $g_k(t,\beta)$ $(k=1,2,\cdots,r)$, we can find the tilted cumulative hazard w_i according to Theorem 3 (with the obvious change of the g functions and number of constraints). Let us denote the resulting tilted cumulative hazard function (with its jumps w_i satisfying (2.38)) as $\Lambda(\beta,t)$.

The maximum empirical likelihood estimator $\hat{\beta}_{MELE}$ satisfies

$$\log EL(\Lambda(\hat{\beta}_{MELE},t)) = \max_{\beta} \log EL(\Lambda(\beta,t)) .$$

Let us define the $r \times r$ matrix Σ with the kl element

$$\Sigma_{kl} = \int \frac{g_k(t,\beta_0)g_l(t,\beta_0)}{[1-F_0(t)][1-G_0(t-)]} d\Lambda_0(t) \tag{2.39}$$

and the $r \times p$ matrix with element

$$B_{kl} = \int \frac{\partial g_k(t,\beta)}{\partial \beta_l} |_{\beta=\beta_0} d\Lambda_0(t) . \tag{2.40}$$

Theorem 15 *Consider the overdetermined hazard estimating equations based on right censored data as given in (2.38). Assume*
(1) The functions $g_k(t,\beta)$ when considered as a function of t are predictable and satisfy the conditions of Theorem 12.
(2) The functions $g_k(t,\beta)$ are twice continuously differentiable in β, for β in a neighborhood of β_0.
(3) The matrix Σ is invertible and the matrix B is full rank.
(4) $\int g_k(t,\beta_0)d\Lambda_0(t) = \mu_k$ for $k = 1,2,\cdots,r$.
Then the empirical likelihood ratio test has asymptotically a chi squared distribution

$$-2[\log EL(\Lambda(\beta_0,t)) - \log EL(\Lambda(\hat{\beta}_{MELE},t)] \xrightarrow{\mathcal{D}} \chi_p^2 ,$$

as $n \to \infty$ under the null hypothesis.

Theorem 16 *Under the same assumptions as in Theorem 15, the maximum empirical likelihood estimator under the overdetermined hazard estimating equations is asymptotically normally distributed as $n \to \infty$.*

$$\sqrt{n}[\hat{\beta}_{MELE} - \beta_0] \xrightarrow{\mathcal{D}} N(0,V) ,$$

where

$$V = \{B^\top \Sigma^{-1} B\}^{-1} .$$

Finally, the matrix B is defined in (2.40).

This maximum empirical likelihood estimator $\hat{\beta}_{MELE}$ also has an optimality property similar to the estimator studied by Qin and Lawless [92].

Theorem 17 *The asymptotic variance of $\hat{\beta}_{MELE}$ does not decease if we drop any one of the estimating equations from r.*

These results are in parallel to those of Qin and Lawless [92]. The difference here is of course that we have right censored data and we use cumulative hazard here (for constructing both the estimating function and the empirical likelihood) instead of distribution functions.

Detailed proofs can be found in Hu [43] and Hu and Zhou [44], which also contain R code for the rank estimator in AFT models and the following example.

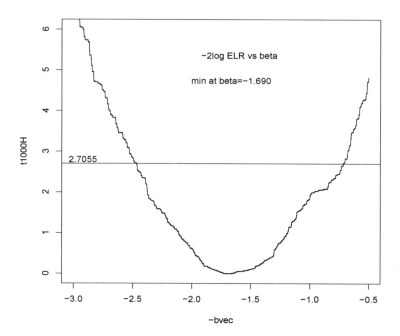

Figure 2.2: The -2LLR vs. β. Just determined case (Gehan).

Example 12 *For the same myeloma data we considered before: if we use* both *the Gehan* and *the log rank estimating functions to form the overdetermined estimating function, we compute* $\hat{\beta} = -1.690$ *and the 90% confidence interval is* $[-2.466, -0.832]$. *Compared to the results before (just-determined case), we see that the estimator is very similar to the Gehan estimator, but the confidence interval here is shorter than either the Gehan or log rank confidence interval, indicating the overdetermined estimator has a smaller variance. If we plot the* -2 *likelihood ratio against* β, *the quadratic-like curve for the just-determined case will be flatter than the overdetermined case near the estimator* $\hat{\beta}$. *The curve is not smooth, indicating the estimating function is not quite continuous with respect to* β. *See Figure 2.2.*

Example 13 *In this example, the right censored data is generated from* $X_i \sim exp(0.02)$ *and* $C_i \sim exp(0.005)$. *The empirical likelihood ratio is smooth with respect to the parameter.*

The two estimating equations with a single parameter θ *are*

$$\int I[0 \le t \le 20] d\Lambda(t) = \theta \tag{2.41}$$

Overdetermined estimating equations

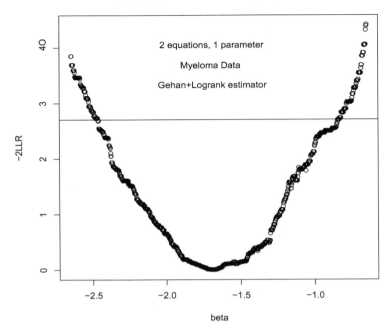

Figure 2.3: The -2LLR vs. β. Overdetermined case.

$$\int I[20 \leq t \leq 40]d\Lambda(t) = \theta. \tag{2.42}$$

Both equations are valid when $\theta = 0.4$ and the true cumulative hazard function equals $0.2t$. We generated a sample of size $n = 100$ and applied either of the two estimating equations above as the constraints (Fig. 2.4). We plot the resulting -2 log empirical likelihood ratio as a function of θ (solid line and dash line). Finally, we use both estimating equations together (as two constraints) and also compute the -2 *log empirical likelihood ratio as a function of θ (line with small circles).*

We see from the plot two things: (1) the minimum locations of the three curves are the three estimators. The three estimators are close to each other. The overdetermined estimator is sandwiched between the two regular estimators. (2) The curvature of the overdetermined case is larger than either one of the just-determined cases. In other words, the overdetermined curve (with circles) has the largest second derivatives at the minimum value. We recall the reciprocal of the second derivative is related to the variance of the estimator.

This second point also leads to a shorter confidence interval: recall the confidence interval obtained by inverting the empirical likelihood ratio test is

$$\{b \mid -2\log ELR(b) \leq \chi_p^2(\alpha)\} .$$

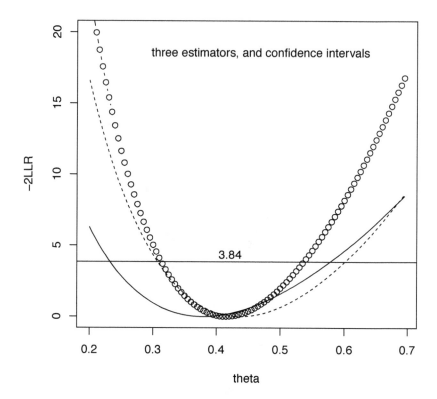

Figure 2.4: Three -2 log empirical likelihood ratios vs. parameter θ.

In the plot we have drawn a horizontal line at 3.84 which is $\chi_1^2(0.95)$. The θ values whose corresponding -2 log likelihood ratio falls below 3.84 form the confidence interval. It is obvious that the confidence interval based on the overdetermined likelihood ratio is shorter than those confidence intervals from either one of the just-determined cases.

2.8   Empirical Likelihood, Binomial Version

The Poisson likelihood we defined in Chapter 1 and used in previous sections has received some criticism. We assumed a discrete hazard/distribution function at some places but at the same time we used a formula connecting the hazard and CDF that is only valid for the continuous case $1 - F(t) = \exp(-\Lambda(t))$.

The binomial version of the censored data empirical likelihood sticks with discrete distribution throughout. If we use the binomial version of empirical likelihood as discussed in Chapter 1, we have parallel results to those with Poisson empirical likelihood. However, the integration of the hazard that defines the parameter takes an unfamiliar form.

Due to the similarity to the results of Poisson empirical likelihood, we state the empirical likelihood results without much proof. For details, the reader may consult the references listed.

Based on the right censored observations, the log empirical likelihood pertaining to a distribution $F(t)$ is

$$\log EL(F) = \sum_i [\delta_i \log \Delta F(T_i) + (1 - \delta_i) \log\{1 - F(T_i)\}] . \qquad (2.43)$$

Since the maximization of the EL will force the distribution to be discrete, we shall use the discrete formula connecting F to the hazard Λ. The equivalent hazard formulation of (2.43) will be denoted by $\log EL(\Lambda)$. Using the relations

$$\Delta\Lambda(t) = \frac{\Delta F(t)}{1 - F(t-)} \quad \text{and} \quad 1 - F(t) = \prod_{s \le t}[1 - \Delta\Lambda(s)] ,$$

we have

$$\log EL = \sum_i \{\delta_i \log(\Delta\Lambda(T_i) \prod_{s < T_i}[1 - \Delta\Lambda(s)]) + (1 - \delta_i) \log(\prod_{s \le T_i}[1 - \Delta\Lambda(s)])\} .$$

We can rewrite this empirical likelihood (proof as homework) as follows. Denoting the jump of the hazard $\Delta\Lambda(T_i) = v_i$, the log EL is given as follows:

$$\log EL(\Lambda) = \sum_i \{d_i \log v_i + (R_i - d_i) \log(1 - v_i)\} , \qquad (2.44)$$

where $d_i = \sum_{j=1}^n I[T_j = t_i]\delta_j$; $R_i = \sum_{j=1}^n I[T_j \ge t_i]$ and t_i are the ordered, distinct values of T_i. The summation in (2.44) runs through all the index of the t_i's. This notation allows the possibility of tied observations.

Thomas and Grunkemeier [112] and Li [67] derived and used the same log empirical likelihood function as (2.44). We shall call this EL the binomial version of the hazard empirical likelihood.

Here, $0 < v_i \le 1$ are the discrete hazards at t_i. The only place v_i may equal 1 is at the largest observed value (and when it is a failure). If $v_i = 1$, then d_i must be positive and $(R_i - d_i)$ must be zero and the term $(R_i - d_i) \log(1 - v_i)$ should be interpreted as zero. If the largest observation is a censored one, then the corresponding $d_i = 0$ and $v_i = 0$ naturally, which makes the log likelihood contribution also zero. Therefore, we may always exclude the largest t_i from the log likelihood computation.

The maximization of (2.44) with respect to v_i is known to be attained at the jumps of the Nelson–Aalen estimator $v_i = d_i/R_i$ by an easy calculation. We further denote the maximum value achieved as $\log EL(\hat{\Lambda}_{NA})$. Notice the similarity of this likelihood to the likelihood of a binomial sample, hence the name.

Let us consider a hypothesis testing problem for a p dimensional parameter defined by

$$\int g_r(t) \log(1 - d\Lambda(t)), \quad \text{for } r = 1, 2, \cdots, p, \qquad (2.45)$$

where the $g_r(t)$ are given functions.

The strange looking parameters defined above could also be written as

$$\int g_r(t)d\log\{1 - F(t)\}, \quad r = 1, 2, \cdots, p.$$

In the continuous case $-\log\{1 - F(t)\}$ *is* the cumulative hazard function, but in the EL analysis, we mainly deal with the discrete case and in the discrete case $-\log\{1 - F(t)\}$ is no longer the cumulative hazard.

The above equivalent formulation is found by using the identity

$$1 - F(t) = \prod_{s \leq t}(1 - d\Lambda(s))$$

and thus we have $d\log\{1 - F(t)\} = \log\{1 - d\Lambda(t)\}$, which, we may check, holds for both discrete *and continuous* $F(t)$. Again, the point t where $F(t) = 1$ has to be excluded from the integration.

The hypothesis we shall consider here is

$$H_0 : \int g_r(s)\log(1 - d\Lambda(s)) = \mu_r \quad \text{for} \quad r = 1, 2, \cdots, p,$$

where μ_r are given constants.

Example 14 *If we take* $g(t) = I[t < a]$, *then* $\int g(t)d\log\{1 - F(t)\} = \log\{1 - F(a-)\}$.

In this example we reproduce the results of Thomas and Grunkemier [112].

We test the probability of survival at least 20 weeks for the second group is 0.7. Another way to formulate this hypothesis is $\log[P(T \geq 20)] = \int I[t < 20]d\log\{1 - F(t)\} = \log(0.7)$.

```
library(emplik)
library(KMsurv)
data(drug6mp)
x=drug6mp$t2
d=drug6mp$relaps
fun4 <- function(x, theta){as.numeric(x < theta)}
emplikH.disc(x=x,d=d,K=log(0.7),fun=fun4,theta=20)
```

The following calculation reproduces the 90% confidence intervals with the 6MP data, sample 2, in Thomas and Grunkemier [112]. For survival probability at 10 weeks.

```
myULfun2 <- function(par, x, d){
                emplikH.disc(x=x, d=d, K=log(par),
                fun=fun4, theta=10)}
findUL(fun=myULfun2, MLE=0.75, level=2.7, x=x, d=d)
## $Low
```

```
## [1] 0.5766238
##
## $Up
## [1] 0.8848779
##
## $FstepL
## [1] 1e-10
##
## $FstepU
## [1] 1e-10
##
## $Lvalue
## [1] 2.7
##
## $Uvalue
## [1] 2.7
```

The default level is 3.84, which corresponds to a 95% confidence interval.

```
findUL(fun=myULfun, MLE=0.75, x=x, d=d)
## $Low
## [1] 0.5401536
##
## $Up
## [1] 0.9037062
##
## $FstepL
## [1] 1e-10
##
## $FstepU
## [1] 1e-10
##
## $Lvalue
## [1] 3.84
##
## $Uvalue
## [1] 3.84
```

This shows the 90% and 95% confidence intervals for $P(T \geq 10)$ are [0.5766238, 0.8848779] *and* [0.5401536, 0.9037062], *respectively.*

What about the ratio/difference of two survival probabilities? We address this in the examples in a later chapter.

The likelihood ratio test statistic calls for the calculation of two empirical likeli-hoods: one (log) EL, maximized with the above null hypothesis constrains, one without. As pointed out, the maximum value of the binomial version of the log empirical likelihood is achieved when there are no constraints by setting $\Lambda(t) = \hat{\Lambda}_{NA}(t)$.

When computing the maximum of the empirical likelihood under the null hypothesis, we again restrict our attention to the hazards that are purely discrete and have jumps only at the observed times. The constraints we shall impose on the discrete hazards v_i are, for given functions $g_1(\cdot),\cdots,g_p(\cdot)$ and constants $\mu_1,\cdots,\mu_p$, we have

$$\sum_{i=1}^{N-1} g_1(t_i)\log(1-v_i) = \mu_1 , \quad \cdots \quad , \quad \sum_{i=1}^{N-1} g_p(t_i)\log(1-v_i) = \mu_p , \qquad (2.46)$$

where N is the total number of distinct observed survival times in the sample. We need to and did exclude the last value as per previous discussion.

Let us abbreviate the maximum likelihood estimators of $\Delta\Lambda(t_i)$ under constraints (2.46) as v_i^*. An application of the Lagrange multiplier method shows that

$$v_i^* = v_i(\lambda) = \frac{d_i}{R_i + n\lambda^\top G(t_i)} , \qquad (2.47)$$

where $G(t_i) = \{g_1(t_i),\cdots,g_p(t_i)\}^T$, and $\lambda = \{\lambda_1,\cdots,\lambda_p\}$ is the root of the p equations

$$\sum_{i=1}^{N-1} g_r(t_i)\log(1 - \frac{d_i}{R_i + n\lambda^\top G(t_i)}) = \mu_r , \quad r = 1,2,\cdots,p. \qquad (2.48)$$

Then the likelihood ratio test statistic for the hypothesis above in terms of hazards is given by

$$\begin{aligned} W_2 &= -2\{\log\max_{v_i} EL(\Lambda)(\text{with constraint } (2.46)) - \log EL(\hat{\Lambda}_{NA})\} \\ &= -2\{\log EL(v_i^*) - \log EL(\hat{\Lambda}_{NA})\} . \end{aligned} \qquad (2.49)$$

We have the following result that is a version of Wilks' theorem for W_2. The regularity conditions include the standard conditions on censoring that allow the Nelson–Aalen estimators to have an asymptotic normal distribution (see, e.g., Andersen et al. [3]) with finite variance.

The proof of the following theorem, along with a detailed set of conditions, can be found in the reference papers.

Theorem 18 *Let $(T_1,\delta_1),\cdots,(T_n,\delta_n)$ be n pairs of i.i.d. observations representing the right censored survival times. Here the survival time distribution $F_0(t)$ may be discrete but $F_0(t)$ and $G_0(t)$ do not jump at the same time. Suppose that the null hypothesis H_0 holds, i.e., $\mu_r = \int g_r(t)\log\{1-d\Lambda_0(t)\}$, $r = 1,2,\cdots,p$. Then, under the regularity conditions that ensure the consistency and asymptotic normality of the Nelson–Aalen integrals $\int g_r(t)\log\{1-d\hat{\Lambda}_{NA}(t)\}$, we have*

$$W_2 \xrightarrow{\mathcal{D}} \chi_p^2$$

as n goes to infinity.

Remark: One of the regularity conditions for Theorem 18 is that the variance-covariance matrix Σ of Nelson–Aalen integrals is invertible. If all elements of Σ are finite yet it is not invertible, then the p constraints may have redundancy within (for example, two identical constraints), in which case we may delete some constraints to make sure the remaining ones are functionally independent.

Remark: Similar to Section 2.5, the functions $g_r(t)$ in the above theorem may be random and depend on n, in which case we require these functions to be predictable with respect to the filtration $\mathcal{F}_t = \sigma\{T_i I_{[T_i \leq t]}; \ \delta_i I_{[T_i \leq t]}; \ i = 1, \ldots, n\}$, plus some convergence properties similar to those in Theorem 12. Then Theorem 18 is still valid.

2.9 Poisson or Binomial?

For a given problem, how shall we chose between the Poisson empirical likelihood and binomial likelihood? We identify two key ingredients affecting the choice: (1) the continuous/discrete nature of the underlying population distribution, (2) how the null hypothesis is laid out, i.e., whether the hypothesis is specified as in (2.5) and Theorem 3 or described in (2.46), (2.47) and (2.48).

Fang [26] carried out extensive simulations to check how well the chi square distribution approximates the null distribution of the -2 log empirical likelihood ratio under various setups. We summarize the basic findings here.

First, if the population is discrete (even if it is created by rounding), then the binomial likelihood is the one to use, and the chi square approximation is adequate. On the other hand, the Poisson log likelihood ratio does not follow the chi square distribution under the null hypothesis, even after we (artificially) break the ties.

Second, if the population is continuous, both the binomial and the Poisson likelihood ratios have good chi square approximation under the null hypothesis. The binomial likelihood ratio may need a slightly larger sample size to achieve good approximation. This is summarized in Table 2.2.

For the setup where the chi square approximation works well for the null distribution, a sample size of 30 seems adequate, unless the NPMLE of the parameter under testing involves the tail of the hazard/survival, which needs larger sample sizes.

Another issue to consider is that the null hypothesis or constraint in the form of log integral (2.46) is rarely used unless the weight function is a simple indicator function. So we try to use the null hypothesis of (2.5) and Theorem 3 whenever possible.

Indeed, if the population distribution is continuous, then both approaches work fine: use either (1) the Poisson EL with the null hypothesis laid out in (2.5) and Theorems 3 and 4; or (2) the binomial EL with the null hypothesis laid out in (2.46) and Theorem 18. The limiting distribution for the log EL ratio test will both be chi square. In fact, the difference between the two likelihood ratio tests converges to zero in probability. See Pan and Zhou [84] for a proof of this fact.

Table 2.2: The Choice of Two Versions of EL and Type of Survival Distribution

Population	Poisson EL	Binomial EL
Continuous	Yes	Yes
Discrete	No	Yes

2.10   Some Notes on Counting Process Martingales

This section is somewhat independent of the rest of materials in this chapter and more heuristic in nature. The martingale constructed from the counting process is used in key places (e.g. Lemma 6) and has become a standard tool in modern survival analysis.

For an arbitrary continuous positive random variable T, the counting process $I[t \geq T]$, for $t > 0$, has one and only one jump of size $+1$, at location $t = T$.

We shall try to identify this one-jump counting process with a transformed Poisson process. The transformations are (1) time acceleration/deceleration and (2) jump size change (increase or decrease).

Mathematically, the two changes are

$$\int_0^t g_2(s)dN(g(s)) \tag{2.50}$$

where $N(t)$ is a standard Poisson process (i.e., with intensity $\equiv 1$), $g(s)$ is a monotone increase function representing a time or clock change and $g_2(s)$ is a function to control the size of the jumps.

If the original Poisson process $N(t)$ has jump times $u_1, u_2, u_3, \cdots$, then it is not hard to see that $N(g(t))$ has jump times $T_1 = g^{-1}(u_1), T_2 = g^{-1}(u_2), \cdots$. Here $g^{-1}(t)$ denotes the inverse function of $g(t)$. Furthermore, the jump sizes of the process (2.50) are $g_2(T_1), g_2(T_2), \cdots$.

A Web page with applet where you can interactively do the time change $(g(s))$ and the jump size change $(g_2(s))$ of a standard Poisson process is available at

http://www.ms.uky.edu/~mai/java/stat/countpro.html

In Fig. 2.5, the two lines we plotted are (1) $\int_0^t g_2(s)dg(s)$, the continuous line, and (2) the random process (2.50), the pure jump line. They are chasing each other. We can control the continuous function by changing $g(t)$ and $g_2(t)$ values. The random jump process will try to follow. In fact, the difference of the two is a martingale process. In the beginning one sixth of time in Fig. 2.5, we did not do anything so that part is just a Poisson process. This is followed by a period with decreased jump size, etc.

Example: Write down a process similar to the Poisson process $N(t)$, except the jump sizes are $1, 1/2, 1/3, 1/4, \cdots$. Solution:

$$\int_0^t \frac{1}{1 + N(s-)} dN(s) \, .$$

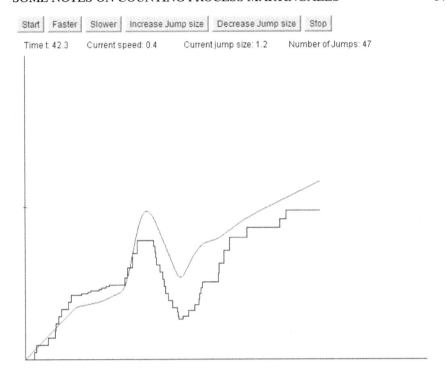

Figure 2.5: Time changed and jump size changed Poisson process and its intensity function.

Here the jump size function $g_2(t) = 1/(1 + N(t-))$ is random but only depends on the history, i.e., predictable. In other words, the value of $g_2(t)$ is determined given the sample path of $N(s)$ for s in $[0,t)$.

Remark: The jump size function $g_2(s)$ and time change function $g(s)$ not only can be fixed functions but can also depend on the history of the process, and still make the game fair, i.e., a martingale. See the next subsection. In the applet of the web page above, this means you may decide how to change $g(s)$ and/or $g_2(s)$ *after* you see the history trajectory of the process. Still, the difference of the two lines in the above applet has mean zero (martingale).

Our next goal is to pick $g(s)$ and $g_2(s)$ functions so that (2.50) mimics the one jump counting process $I[t \geq T]$. We shall see that $g(s)$ will be a fixed function and $g_2(s)$ actually only depends on the history.

First, since the waiting time of the first jump of a Poisson process is a random variable with an exponential distribution, and the jump time of $I[t \geq T]$ is T, we need a function $g(s)$ to change the exponential distribution to the distribution $F_T(t) = P(T \leq t)$.

Theorem 19 *Assume T is a continuous random variable. If $g(s) = $ cumulative hazard function of T, then the waiting time for the first jump of the process $N(g(s))$ is a random variable with distribution $F_T(t) = P(T \leq t)$.*

PROOF: Denote the first jump time of the process $N(g(s))$ by T_1, then

$$P(T_1 > t) = P(N(g(t)) = 0) = \exp(-g(t))$$

by the Poisson assumption of the $N(t)$. Since $g(t) = H_T(t)$, we have

$$\exp(-g(t)) = \exp(-H_T(t)) = 1 - F_T(t),$$

because $H_T(t)$ is continuous. □

Second, in order for (2.50) to mimic $I[t \geq T]$, the function $g_2(s)$ needs to keep the first jump size of the (now time changed) Poisson process unchanged (since both processes have jumps of size 1), but any subsequent jumps of the (time changed) Poisson process need to be shrunk down to size zero (i.e., no jumps other than the first one). This implies that $g_2(s)$ should take the value 1 all the way up to and including the first jump time T_1 but zero afterwards: $g_2(s) = I[s \leq T_1]$, where T_1 is the time of the first jump of $N(g(t))$. By the above theorem, T_1 has the same distribution as T.

Combining the above two points, we have the following theorem.

Theorem 20 *The one jump counting process $I[t \geq T]$ is equivalent in distribution to $\int_0^t I[s \leq T_1] dN(g(s))$, with $g(s) = H_T(s)$. We also have T_1 (the first jump time of the process $N(g(s))$) equal in distribution to T.*

2.10.1 Compensated Counting Process as Martingale

If $N(t)$ is a standard Poisson process, then it is easy to verify

$$N(t) - t = M(t)$$

is a martingale in t.

Remark: To be rigorous, we need to specify the increasing family of σ algebra of events $\mathcal{F}_t$ and verify the conditional expectation in order to claim the $M(t)$ above to be a martingale. But our exposition here is informal and intended to be intuitive, so we are not going through the definition-theorem-proof-corollary cycle. We shall be satisfied to say that since the Poisson process has independent increments, therefore the required conditional expectation to verify the martingale claim is the same as an unconditional expectation and thus can be verified easily (using memoryless property) to be zero.

After a time change (from t to $g(t)$), the following is also a martingale:

$$N(g(t)) - g(t) = M(g(t)) .$$

Notice that we need to require the time change $g(t)$ to be a fixed function or predictable, so that in the verification of the martingale conditional expectation it acts like a fixed function.

It is not too hard to verify the mean of the process $\int_0^t g_2(s)dN(g(s))$ is

$$\int_0^t g_2(s)dg(s) ,$$

and the variance of the process $\int_0^t g_2(s)dN(g(s))$ is

$$\int_0^t [g_2(s)]^2 dg(s) .$$

Also,

$$\int_0^t g_2(s)dN(g(s)) - \int_0^t g_2(s)dg(s)$$

is a martingale, and its predictable variation ("variance") process is

$$\int_0^t [g_2(s)]^2 dg(s) .$$

These should be easy to verify when $g_2(s)$ and $g(s)$ are fixed functions. (Further simplification is possible if we assume $g_2(t)$ is piecewise constant.) A little further investigation will convince us that they can both be predictable functions. The predictable variation process of a martingale $M(t)$ is usually denoted by $\langle M(t) \rangle$.

Using the above calculations, we finally have

$$\begin{aligned} M(t) &= \int_0^t I[s \leq T_1]d\{N(g(s)) - g(s)\} \\ &= \int_0^t I[s \leq T_1]dN(g(s)) - \int_0^t I[s \leq T_1]dg(s), \end{aligned}$$

which is also a martingale, since $g_2(s) = I[s \leq T_1]$ is clearly predictable.

Using the above theorem, we see that

$$I[t \geq T] - \int_0^t I[s \leq T]dg(s) = I[t \geq T] - \int_0^t I[s \leq T]h_T(s)ds \qquad (2.51)$$

is a martingale, where the second equality is due to the fact that $g(s)$ is the cumulative hazard function of T, as required by the above theorem.

Example: The process that has jump sizes $1, 1/2, 1/3, 1/4, \cdots$ can be made into a martingale. Solution:

$$\int_0^t \frac{1}{1+N(s-)}dN(s) - \int_0^t \frac{1}{1+N(s-)}ds = M(t) .$$

2.10.2   Censoring as Splitting/Thinning of a Counting Process

Recall that we may split a Poisson process by further classifying its jumps as one of several types. A similar thing also works here for the one jump process $I[t \geq T]$. The two types of jumps we classify here will be censored/uncensored.

Let $X > 0$ be the failure time and $C > 0$ be the censoring time. Assume they are independent. Let $T = \min(X, C)$.

The counting process based on T is $N^+(t) = I[t \geq T]$. The intensity for this (one-jump) counting process is $h_T(t)I[T \geq t]$ (i.e., $I[t \geq T] - \int_0^t h_T(s)I[T \geq s]ds$ is a martingale by (2.51)).

Censoring is to split the event of jumping into two types, either a failure type or a censoring type, indicated by the value $\delta = I[X \leq C] = I[T = X]$.

After splitting, we have two counting processes, $N^x(t) = I[T \leq t, \delta = 1]$ and $N^c(t) = I[T \leq t, \delta = 0]$. They also have splitting intensities: $h_x(t)I[T \geq t]$ and $h_c(t)I[T \geq t]$, respectively. Here we denote the hazard function of the random variable C as $h_c(t)$, the hazard of X as $h_x(t)$, etc.

Notice we have

$$N^x(t) + N^c(t) = N^+(t) = I[T \leq t]$$

and also

$$h_x(t)I[T \geq t] + h_c(t)I[T \geq t] = h_T(t)I[T \geq t].$$

The last equality is true since $T = \min(X, C)$ and X is independent of C.

To summarize, we have three counting process martingales:

$$M(t) = I[T \leq t] - \int_0^t I[T \geq s]h_T(s)ds$$

$$M^x(t) = I[T \leq t, \delta = 1] - \int_0^t I[T \geq s]h_x(s)ds \qquad (2.52)$$

and

$$M^c(t) = I[T \leq t, \delta = 0] - \int_0^t I[T \geq s]h_c(s)ds .$$

The second martingale, $M^x(t)$, is the one that we use in survival analysis most often.

2.11   Discussion, Remarks, and Historical Notes

Pan and Zhou [84] is the main reference for this chapter. They also explicitly gave the feasible region for λ. For the special case of $g(t) = I[t \leq a]$, the hazard empirical likelihood was also considered by Murphy [74].

Zhou [137] also studied the rank estimating equations for AFT models, but there the empirical likelihood was formulated in terms of the Kaplan–Meier estimator instead of the hazard function. He did not consider the overdetermined case.

Counting processes have become an indispensable part of modern survival analysis since the pioneering work of Aalen [1]. The theory and applications are summarized in Fleming and Harrington [28] and Andersen et al. [3].

However, even within an advanced survival analysis course, these two books are too huge. Both counting process books mentioned above are over 400 pages. Kalbfleisch and Prentice [51], Chapter 5, is more manageable. We offer here a quick and simple interpretation of the counting process martingales presuming only knowledge of Poisson processes. The treatment here is heuristic and only for continuous random variables but should satisfy many survival analysis courses for a quick introduction of the topic.

For right censored data, Naik-Nimbalkar and Rajarshi [76] discussed the use of empirical likelihood to test if the k independent samples have equal medians. They also defined an estimator of the common median under the null hypothesis. This is actually a case of the overdetermined EL estimator, since under the null hypothesis, the true median can be estimated from any of the k samples. See Example 17 in Chapter 3.

2.12   Exercises

Exercise 2.1 *Show that the empirical likelihood expression just before (2.44) can be simplified to (2.44).*

Exercise 2.2 *The mean and variance of the standard Poisson process at time t is t. What is the mean of the pure jump process $N(g(t))$? What about the process $\int_0^t g_2(s)dN(g(s))$? [First assume $g_2(s)$ is a piecewise constant function.] What is the conditional mean of the increment of this process? Does it have independent increments?*

Exercise 2.3 *Suppose X and C are two independent, positive random variables. Assume both of them have densities. Let $\delta = I[X < C]$. Given that the minimum value of X and C is t, show that the probability that the value t coming from X, $P(\delta = 1 | \min(X,C) = t)$, is*

$$\frac{h_x(t)}{h_x(t) + h_c(t)} .$$

This is the splitting probability, when a jump at time t in the variable T occurs.

Exercise 2.4 *Verify Lemma 8.*

Exercise 2.5 *Verify that the predictable variation process of the martingale*

$$M^x(t) = I[T \le t, \delta = 1] - \int_0^t I[T \ge s]h_x(s)ds$$

is

$$\int_0^t I[T \ge s]h_x(s)ds .$$

Exercise 2.6 *In the context of Example 10, fit a Cox model to the data* smallcell, *using only* arm *as a covariate. Compare the p-value from the score test to the log rank test obtained by* survdiff( ).

Exercise 2.7 *The following code will generate two samples of observations. Sample one has a constant hazard λ_1 (exponential random variable). Sample two initially has a high hazard (higher than λ_1) but as t increases, the hazard decreases to a level that is lower than λ_1. This might represent a treatment that has a good long-term effect but is risky in the short-term.*

```
cumhazfun <- function(t, a=0.2, b=0.8){a*t + b*(1-exp(-t))}
invhazfun <- function(y, fun=cumhazfun){
              myhazfun1 <- function(t){fun(t) - y}
              temp <- uniroot(f=myhazfun1, lower=-0.1,
                              upper=100)
              return(temp$root)
}
rvgenerate <- function(n=1){
              temp <- rexp(n)
              for(i in 1:n) temp[i] <- invhazfun(y=temp[i])
              return(temp)
}
```

Let us now generate two samples of observations with hazard $h_1(t) = 0.3$ and $h_2(t) = 0.2 + 0.8e^{-t}$, respectively.

```
ft1 <- rexp(100)/0.3
ft2 <- rvgenerate(100)
cen1 <- rexp(100)/0.1
cen2 <- rexp(100)/0.12
status1 <- as.numeric(cen1 >= ft1)
status2 <- as.numeric(cen2 >= ft2)
obs1 <- pmin(ft1, cen1)
obs2 <- pmin(ft2, cen2)
```

Verify that the log rank test has low power detecting the difference for the above two samples: (obs1, status1) *and* (obs2, status2).

Use this generated data and re-run Example 10. Compare the power of the log rank test and the combined test.

Chapter 3

Empirical Likelihood for Linear Functionals of the Cumulative Distribution Function

In this chapter we study the empirical likelihood test and the associated Wilks theorem for right censored data when the hypotheses are formulated in terms of p linear functionals of the CDF. These hypotheses or parameters can also be described by p estimating equations or mean functions.

In particular, we show that the log empirical likelihood ratio test statistic is equal to a quadratic form similar to Hotelling's T^2 statistic, plus a small error. The least favorable distribution is given explicitly in terms of advanced time transformation of the density. An alternative proof is also discussed.

3.1 One-Sample Means

We first introduce some notation and formulate the basic setup. The main theorem of this chapter is Theorem 23. Some tedious calculations are appended afterwards.

Suppose that $X_1, X_2, \cdots, X_n$ are i.i.d. nonnegative random variables denoting lifetimes, with a continuous distribution function F_0. Independent of the lifetimes, there are censoring times $C_1, C_2, \ldots, C_n$, which are i.i.d. with a distribution G_0. Only the observations (T_i, δ_i) are available to us, where

$$T_i = \min(X_i, C_i) \quad \text{and} \quad \delta_i = I[X_i \leq C_i] \quad \text{for } i = 1, 2, \cdots, n.$$

Remark: The identical distribution assumption on the censoring time C_i is not essential. In many cases, the requirement of i.i.d. censoring times with CDF $G_0(t)$ can be replaced by independent censoring with CDF $G_{0i}(t)$ and some requirements on the average CDF $1/n \sum_{i=1}^{n} G_{0i}(t)$. Since the conditions are much simpler to describe for an i.i.d. setting, we shall retain the i.i.d. assumption.

The empirical likelihood of censored data in terms of distribution (see discussion in Chapter 1 or Owen [81] (6.9)) is defined as

$$EL(F) \quad = \quad \prod_{i=1}^{n} [\Delta F(T_i)]^{\delta_i} [1 - F(T_i)]^{1-\delta_i} \tag{3.1}$$

$$= \prod_{i=1}^{n}[\Delta F(T_i)]^{\delta_i}\{\sum_{j:T_j>T_i}\Delta F(T_j)\}^{1-\delta_i} \qquad (3.2)$$

where $\Delta F(t) = F(t) - F(t-)$ is the jump of F at t. The second line above assumes a discrete $F(\cdot)$ with possible jumps at T_i only. Letting $w_i = \Delta F(T_i)$ for $i = 1, 2, \cdots, n$, the likelihood for this discrete F can then be written in terms of the jumps as

$$EL = \prod_{i=1}^{n}[w_i]^{\delta_i}\{\sum_{j=1}^{n} w_j I[T_j > T_i]\}^{1-\delta_i} ,$$

and the log likelihood is

$$\log EL = \sum_{i=1}^{n}\left\{ \delta_i \log w_i + (1-\delta_i)\log \sum_{j=1}^{n} w_j I[T_j > T_i]\right\} . \qquad (3.3)$$

If we maximize the log EL above without constraint (i.e., no extra constraints; the probability constraint $w_i \geq 0, \sum w_i = 1$ is always imposed), it is well-known that the Kaplan–Meier estimator [52], $w_i = \Delta \hat{F}_{KM}(T_i)$, achieves the maximum value of the log EL.

Kiefer and Wolferwitz [53] defined a nonparametric maximum likelihood estimator, where there is no σ-finite dominating measure on the family of the densities under consideration, and they showed that the empirical distribution function is a nonparametric maximum likelihood estimator of the CDF for i.i.d. observations. Li [67] showed that for right censored data the empirical likelihood we discuss here can also be viewed as the nonparametric likelihood of Kiefer and Wolferwitz. Thus the Kaplan–Meier estimator is indeed a nonparametric maximum likelihood estimator per the Kiefer and Wolferwitz definition.

Similar arguments to Owen [78] show that we may restrict our attention in the EL analysis (i.e., the search for a maximum under the null hypothesis) to discrete CDFs F that are dominated by the Kaplan–Meier estimator $F(t) \ll \hat{F}_{KM}(t)$. Owen [78] restricted his attention to those distribution functions F that are dominated by the empirical distribution. Intuitively, the maximization forces the distribution to be discrete.

To form the ratio of two empirical likelihoods, we not only need to find the maximum of log EL among all F (which is achieved by the Kaplan–Meier estimator), but we also need to find the maximum of log EL under a null hypothesis. Here we shall use the popular null hypothesis involving linear functionals of the CDF or mean functionals. As Owen [78] has shown, this includes the M- and Z- estimates.

The next step in our analysis is to find a discrete CDF, F, that maximizes log $EL(F)$ under null hypothesis (3.4) or (3.5), which are specified as follows:

$$\int_{0}^{\infty} g_1(t)dF(t) = \mu_1$$

$$\int_{0}^{\infty} g_2(t)dF(t) = \mu_2 \qquad (3.4)$$

$$\cdots \quad \cdots$$

$$\int_0^\infty g_p(t)dF(t) = \mu_p$$

where $g_i(t)\, i = 1, 2, \ldots, p$ are given functions that satisfy some moment conditions (specified later), and $\mu_i\, i = 1, 2, \ldots, p$ are given constants. Without loss of generality, we shall assume all $\mu_i = 0$. The constraints (3.4) can be written, for a discrete CDF, with $w_i = \Delta F(T_i)$, as

$$\sum_{i=1}^n g_1(T_i)w_i = 0$$

$$\sum_{i=1}^n g_2(T_i)w_i = 0 \qquad\qquad (3.5)$$

$$\cdots \quad \cdots$$

$$\sum_{i=1}^n g_p(T_i)w_i = 0 \,.$$

Remark: The null hypothesis

$$\int g(t)dF(t) = \mu$$

looks similar to those we considered in Chapter 2,

$$\int g(t)d\Lambda(t) = \theta \,,$$

yet there is a critical difference. Using the relation between hazard function and distribution function, we have

$$\int g(t)d\Lambda(t) = \int g(t)\frac{dF(t)}{1 - F(t-)} \,. \qquad\qquad (3.6)$$

If $1 - F(t-)$ in the denominator of the right-hand side above can be considered *fixed* when finding the constrained maximum of the empirical likelihood function with respect to F, then (3.6) is just a mean constraint. However, the hazard constraint (3.6) is such that the two F's on the right-hand side of (3.6) must change simultaneously to satisfy the constraint and to maximize the empirical likelihood function. On the other hand, if the hazard constraint were

$$\int g(t)\exp[-\Lambda(t)]d\Lambda(t) = \theta \,,$$

then the hazard constraints would be asymptotically equivalent to the mean constraint (at least for the continuous F_0).

We must find the maximum of $\log EL(F)$ under these constraints (3.5). We accomplish this in three steps. First, we construct a p-parameter family of CDFs that passes through (and is dominated by) the Kaplan–Meier estimator in the direction h.

We then find the CDF in this family that satisfies the constraints. Finally, we maximize $\log EL$ over all possible h.

Notice that *any* discrete CDF dominated by the Kaplan–Meier estimator can *always* be written (in terms of its jumps) as

$$\Delta F(T_i) = \Delta \hat{F}_{KM}(T_i)[1 - h(T_i)], \quad i = 1, 2, \cdots, n,$$

for *some* h function. Of course this distribution usually does not satisfy the constraints (3.5) above. This motivates us to define the following:

For any p given functions of t, $h = (h_1(t), \cdots, h_p(t))$, we define a family of distributions (indexed by $\lambda \in \mathbb{R}^p$ and dominated by the Kaplan–Meier estimator) by its jumps

$$\Delta F_\lambda(T_i) = \Delta \hat{F}_{KM}(T_i)[1 - \lambda^\top h(T_i)] \tag{3.7}$$

where $\lambda^\top h(T_i)$ is the inner product $\lambda_1 h_1(T_i) + \ldots + \lambda_p h_p(T_i)$ and the total jumps sum to one, as any discrete CDF must. This requirement leads to

$$\sum_i h(T_i) \Delta \hat{F}_{KM}(T_i) = 0. \tag{3.8}$$

Since the jumps of the Kaplan–Meier estimator are between zero and one, therefore at least for small values of λ (in a neighborhood of zero) the jumps of F_λ as defined above will be between zero and one. Thus F_λ is a legitimate distribution for those small λs. Obviously, when $\lambda = 0$, we have $F_{\lambda=0} = \hat{F}_{KM}$.

We shall also, without loss of generality, require that $\|h\|_2 = K$, for some fixed constant $K > 0$ (since we may always have a scale adjustment on λ: $\lambda^\top h = (\lambda/a)^\top ah$). We shall take $\lambda = (\lambda_1, \ldots, \lambda_p)$ as the parameter whose value is selected to make this distribution satisfy the hypothesis/constraints (3.5) above. The requirement that the distribution satisfy the constraints/hypothesis (3.5) will force λ to take certain values, as in the following equation:

$$0 = \sum_{i=1}^{n} g_j(T_i) \Delta F_\lambda(T_i) \quad j = 1, 2, \cdots, p. \tag{3.9}$$

Denote the solution of the above equation as λ^*. The fact that it has a unique solution is guaranteed by the assumption that matrix A (defined in Lemma 22 below) is invertible. (In fact, we will assume a slightly stronger condition: that the condition number of A is *bounded* away from zero.)

The next lemma will be useful later. It is the central limit theorem of the Kaplan–Meier integrals.

Lemma 21 *Define a vector gg of length p with elements*

$$gg_j = \sum_i g_j(T_i) \Delta \hat{F}_{KM}(T_i).$$

Under the null hypothesis, we have (since the true mean of g is assumed to be zero under the null hypothesis, no centering constants are needed)

$$\sqrt{n}\, gg \xrightarrow{\mathcal{D}} N(0, \Sigma) \quad \text{as } n \to \infty.$$

The asymptotic ($p \times p$) variance-covariance matrix $\Sigma = [\sigma_{jk}]$ (assumed to be non-singular) is given by

$$\sigma_{jk} = \int [g_j(x) - \bar{g}_j(x)][g_k(x) - \bar{g}_k(x)] \frac{dF_0(x)}{1 - G_0(x-)}$$

and it can be consistently estimated by $\hat{\Sigma} = [\hat{\sigma}_{jk}]$

$$\hat{\sigma}_{jk} = \sum_{i=1}^{n} [g_j(T_i) - \bar{g}_j(T_i)][g_k(T_i) - \bar{g}_k(T_i)] \frac{\Delta \hat{F}_{KM}(T_i)}{1 - \hat{G}_{KM}(T_i)} ,$$

where $\bar{g}_j$ is the advanced-time transformation of g_j defined by Efron and Johnstone [24], either with respect to F_0 (in σ_{jk} above) or with respect to the Kaplan–Meier estimator (in $\hat{\sigma}_{jk}$ above). See also Lemma 26 in the next section for advanced-time transformation. Finally, $\hat{G}_{KM}$ is the Kaplan–Meier estimator of the censoring distribution.

PROOF: This lemma is just the multivariate asymptotic normality of the Kaplan–Meier integral, which has been treated by many others before. The new part is the variance-covariance formula. It can easily be proved by using the representation results of Akritas [2], which contain a univariate version of this lemma. With the representation one then uses the multivariate central limit theorem for the counting process martingales to finish the proof. One such multivariate central limit theorem for counting process martingales can be found in Kalbfleish and Prentice, Chapter 5 [51].

The assertion that the variance-covariance can be consistently estimated can be seen from the fact that it is a plug-in estimator. □

Solving Equation (3.9) gives the following solution of λ for the constraint equations, which we call λ^*.

Lemma 22 *Let us denote the solution of (3.9) as λ^*. Then the distribution F_λ within the family (3.7) that satisfies the constraint (3.9) must satisfy*

$$\lambda^* A = gg .$$

If the matrix A is invertible, we have

$$\lambda^* = A^{-1} gg$$

where the $p \times p$ matrix $A = [a_{jk}]$ is defined by the elements

$$a_{jk} = \sum_{i=1}^{n} g_j(T_i) h_k(T_i) \Delta \hat{F}_{KM}(T_i) . \tag{3.10}$$

Also, the elements may be written as

$$a_{jk} = \sum_{i} [g_j(T_i) - Eg_j][h_k(T_i) - Eh_k] \Delta \hat{F}_{KM}(T_i) .$$

PROOF: Solve Equation (3.9) to arrive at the stated result. The second expression of a_{jk} is valid since $\sum_i h_k(T_i)\Delta\hat{F}_{KM}(T_i) = 0$, so both of the a_{jk} expressions are valid expressions of the covariance. □

Remark: We are to find the maximum of the $\log EL$ among all h. Yet we placed some restrictions on h. The assumption we need to place on h, for given g, is that this matrix A should be invertible. For those h where A is not invertible, we may argue that this sub-family of distributions does not have a solution that satisfies the constraints (3.5), and thus can be ignored in the search to maximize $\log EL$ *under constraints*. On the other hand, the least favorable h^* we calculated in (3.15) of Lemma 25 will lead to an A matrix that is identical to $\hat{\Sigma}$ defined in Lemma 21, which by assumption is a nonsingular variance-covariance matrix for sufficiently large n, and thus invertible.

Remark: Under the null hypothesis, gg is of order $O_p(1/\sqrt{n})$ (Lemma 21). If the h function is such that the inverse matrix of A has a bounded condition number, then λ^* is also of order $O_p(1/\sqrt{n})$, uniformly for those h.

Remark: In order to work with the inverse matrix, we end up with a condition on h in terms of a matrix as below. We assume the following matrix is positive definite:

$$A^\infty = (a_{ij}^\infty), \quad \text{where} \quad a_{ij}^\infty = \int_0^\infty g_i(t)h_j(t)dF_0(t) . \tag{3.11}$$

Since we assumed this matrix is invertible, as a finite sample version, A should also be invertible for large enough n, as required in Lemma 22. The consequence of this is that we need to avoid those h that are (almost) orthogonal to g. We will see in (3.15) that the particular h we are interested in is not orthogonal to g, in fact, far from it.

We shall call the CDF F_λ defined in (3.7) a tilted Kaplan–Meier distribution. The size of λ controls the amount of tilting, in the direction h. When $\lambda = 0$, there is no tilting and we have $F_{\lambda=0} = \hat{F}_{KM}$.

Define $f(\lambda) = \log EL(F_\lambda)$. The Wilks statistic is then just

$$2[f(0) - \sup_h f(\lambda^*)] = -2\log ELR.$$

Taking a Taylor expansion with $f(\lambda^*)$, we have

$$\text{Wilks statistics} = \inf_h 2\{f(0) - f(0) - \lambda^* f'(0) - 1/2[\lambda^*]^\top f''(0)\lambda^* + O_p(\lambda^*)\}.$$

Notice that $f'(0) = 0$ since the derivative of log likelihood at the maximum (i.e., the Kaplan–Meier estimator) must be zero for any h. Recall the Kaplan–Meier estimator is the MLE that maximizes $\log EL$. This fact can also be readily checked using the self-consistency identity (see Section 3.2) and the fact that $\sum_i h(T_i)\Delta\hat{F}_{KM}(T_i) = 0$.

We finally have

$$\text{Wilks statistics} = \inf_h [\sqrt{n}\lambda^*]^\top \left(-f''(0)/n\right)[\sqrt{n}\lambda^*] + o_p(1), \tag{3.12}$$

where the $o_p(1)$ is uniform over h, which we pointed out is true under the assumption of condition number for the matrix A^∞ (see Remarks after Lemma 22).

The rest of the analysis will focus on the first term on the right-hand side of (3.12) above. First we calculate the second derivative f'' and simplify it. Then we show the infimum over h of the right-hand (ignore the $o_p(1)$ part) is achieved at an h satisfying Equation (3.15) below. And finally, for this particular h, the above Wilks statistic becomes Hotelling's T^2 plus $o_p(1)$ and thus has asymptotically a chi square distribution with degrees of freedom p.

Theorem 23 *Let* $(T_1, \delta_1), \ldots, (T_n, \delta_n)$ *be* n *pairs of i.i.d. censored random variables as defined above. Suppose* g_i $i = 1, \ldots, p$ *are given functions such that the* $p \times p$ *asymptotic variance-covariance matrix of the Kaplan–Meier mean estimator,* $\int g_i(t) d\hat{F}_{KM}(t)$, *is well defined and positive definite. That is, the* $p \times p$ *matrix* Σ *below is well defined and positive definite:*

$$\Sigma = (\sigma_{jk}) = \int \frac{[g_j(x) - \bar{g}_j(x)][g_k(x) - \bar{g}_k(x)]}{(1 - G_0(x-))} dF_0(x) . \qquad (3.13)$$

Then, under null hypothesis (3.4) as $n \to \infty$, *we have*

$$-2 \log ELR \xrightarrow{\;D\;} \chi^2_{(p)} \quad as \quad n \to \infty$$

where $\log ELR = \sup_h \log EL(F_{\lambda*}) - \log EL(\hat{F}_{KM})$.
In fact, we have

$$-2 \log ELR = [\sqrt{n}gg]^{\top} \hat{\Sigma}^{-1} [\sqrt{n}gg] + o_p(1) ,$$

where gg *and* $\hat{\Sigma}$ *are defined in Lemma 21.*

A sufficient condition which will guarantee the (single) integral in (3.13) is well defined was pointed out by Akritas [2]:

$$0 < \int \frac{g_j^2(x)}{1 - G_0(x-)} dF_0(x) < \infty , \quad j = 1, \cdots, p.$$

To ensure the matrix Σ is nonsingular, we require that the g_i functions (p of them) are so-called linearly independent. In other words, the p constraints are all genuine, without redundancy.

The Q–Q plot (Fig. 3.1) confirms the approximate chi square distribution of the $-2 \log$ empirical likelihood ratio under the null hypothesis. When there are more than one mean constraints, or when censoring rate is higher, the chi square approximation needs a larger sample size to take hold.

3.2 Proof of Theorem 23

This section might be skipped on the first reading if the reader's main interest is in possible applications of the empirical likelihood method.

PROOF OF THEOREM 23. We proceed by proving two more lemmas.

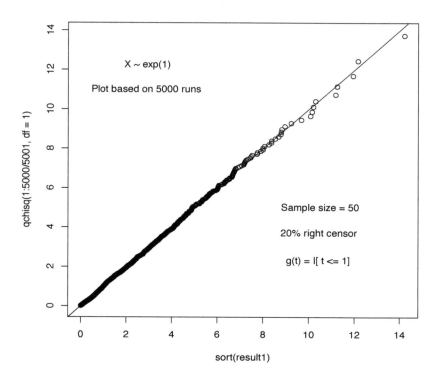

Figure 3.1: Q–Q plot of $-2 \log$ EL ratio under the null hypothesis.

Lemma 24 *The second derivative $f''(0)$ defined in (3.12) above is equal to $-nB$ with the elements of the matrix B defined below in (3.14).*

We now compute the second derivative $f''(0)$. Straightforward calculation shows that this is a $p \times p$ matrix. The jkth elements of matrix $[-f''(0)/n] = B = [b_{jk}]$ are given by

$$
\begin{aligned}
b_{jk} &= \sum_{i=1}^{n} h_j(T_i) h_k(T_i) \frac{\delta_i}{n} \\
&+ \sum_{i=1}^{n} \frac{1-\delta_i}{n} \frac{[\sum_{m:T_m>T_i} h_j(T_m)\Delta\hat{F}_{KM}(T_m)][\sum_{m:T_m>T_i} h_k(T_m)\Delta\hat{F}_{KM}(T_m)]}{[1-\hat{F}_{KM}(T_i)]^2}.
\end{aligned}
$$

After several rounds of tedious simplifications (see below for details), we have

$$
b_{jk} = \sum_{i=1}^{n} [h_j(T_i) - \bar{h}_j(T_i)][h_k(T_i) - \bar{h}_k(T_i)][1-\hat{G}_{KM}(T_i)]\Delta\hat{F}_{KM}(T_i). \qquad (3.14)
$$

Lemma 25 *(Matrix Cauchy–Schwarz inequality)* *For any h we have*

$$[A^{-1}]^\top B A^{-1} \geq \hat{\Sigma}^{-1}$$

where the $\geq$ *means the matrix inequality for positive-definite matrices. And the equality is achieved by* h^* *that satisfies (3.15) below. For* $j = 1, 2, \ldots, p,$

$$[h_j^*(x) - \bar{h}_j^*(x)] = \frac{g_j(x) - \bar{g}_j(x)}{1 - \hat{G}_{KM}(x-)} \qquad a.s. \quad \hat{F}_{KM} . \tag{3.15}$$

Clearly, any h that is a constant multiple of h^* *also satisfies (3.15). (* h^* *has a constant free play.)*

PROOF: First we rewrite the entries of matrix A as

$$a_{jk} = \sum_{i=1}^{n} \frac{g_j(T_i) - \bar{g}_j(T_i)}{\sqrt{1 - \hat{G}_{KM}(T_i)}} [h_k(T_i) - \bar{h}_k(T_i)] \sqrt{1 - \hat{G}_{KM}(T_i)} \, \Delta \hat{F}_{KM}(T_i) .$$

This is valid due to the advanced transformation identity, which we formulate in Lemma 26. So, in terms of the expectation with respect to the Kaplan–Meier estimator, we have

$$a_{jk} = E \frac{(g - \bar{g})}{\sqrt{1 - G}} (h - \bar{h}) \sqrt{1 - G} = E(\alpha\beta), \quad \text{say}$$

and furthermore,

$$b_{jk} = E (h - \bar{h}) \sqrt{1 - G} (h - \bar{h}) \sqrt{1 - G} = E(\beta^2) ,$$

$$\hat{\sigma}_{jk} = E \frac{g - \bar{g}}{\sqrt{1 - G}} \frac{g - \bar{g}}{\sqrt{1 - G}} = E(\alpha^2) .$$

The inequality can then follow easily from the well-known matrix Cauchy–Schwarz inequality (see Tripathi [113] and references therein). □

Using Lemma 25, we see that for any y, the quadratic form have inequality $y^\top [A^{-1}]^\top B A^{-1} y \geq y^\top \hat{\Sigma}^{-1} y$. And the equality is achieved when h satisfies (3.15).

Using Lemmas 21, 22 and 24 and this Cauchy–Schwarz inequality, we see that

$$\text{Wilks Statistics} \quad = \quad \inf_h [\sqrt{n}gg]^\top [A^{-1}]^\top B A^{-1} [\sqrt{n}gg] + o_p(1) \tag{3.16}$$

$$= \quad [\sqrt{n}gg]^\top \hat{\Sigma}^{-1} [\sqrt{n}gg] + o_p(1) .$$

As $n \to \infty$, the right-hand side is clearly converging to a chi square distribution under the null hypothesis with $df = p$. The proof of Theorem 23 is now complete. □

Remark: In other words, the least favorable direction is given by (3.15). Or, if we define a parametric model by Equation (3.15), this is what Stein [105] called the most difficult parametric sub-problem.

Remark: If we want to profile out part of the parameters in the above empirical likelihood ratio, we shall get a chi square distribution with reduced degrees of freedom. This can be easily seen from the asymptotic representation of the empirical likelihood ratio as a Hotelling's T^2, for which the similar profiling result is well-known.

SIMPLIFICATION OF THE SECOND DERIVATIVE $-f''(0)/n$.

The first simplification uses the self-consistency identity (Lemma 27 below, with $g = h_j h_k$) to the first term of $-f''(0)/n$.

$$b_{jk} = \sum_{i=1}^{n} h_j(T_i)h_k(T_i)\Delta\hat{F}_{KM}(T_i) - \sum_{i=1}^{n}\frac{1-\delta_i}{n}\frac{\displaystyle\sum_{T_j>T_i} h_j(T_j)h_k(T_j)\Delta\hat{F}_{KM}(T_j)}{1-\hat{F}_{KM}(T_i)}$$

$$+\sum_{i=1}^{n}\frac{1-\delta_i}{n}\frac{[\displaystyle\sum_{m:T_m>T_i} h_j(T_m)\Delta\hat{F}_{KM}(T_m)][\displaystyle\sum_{m:T_m>T_i} h_k(T_m)\Delta\hat{F}_{KM}(T_m)]}{[1-\hat{F}_{KM}(T_i)]^2}.$$

The last two summations above (those with $1-\delta_i$) can be combined by using the identity $\mathbb{E}XY - (\mathbb{E}X)(\mathbb{E}Y) = \mathbb{E}(X-\mathbb{E}X)(Y-\mathbb{E}Y)$. In fact, we use it n times, each with a different conditional distribution, to get the following:

$$b_{jk} = \sum_{i=1}^{n} h_j(T_i)h_k(T_i)\Delta\hat{F}_{KM}(T_i) -$$

$$\sum_{i=1}^{n}\frac{1-\delta_i}{n}\frac{\displaystyle\sum_{m:T_m>T_i}[h_j(T_m)-E_{\hat{F}}(h_j|t>T_i)][h_k(T_m)-E_{\hat{F}}(h_k|t>T_i)]\Delta\hat{F}_{KM}(T_m)}{1-\hat{F}_{KM}(T_i)}.$$

Notice we have many expressions of covariances in the second term above. The first summation can also be written as $\sum[h_j-\mathbb{E}h_j][h_k-\mathbb{E}h_k]\Delta\hat{F}_{KM}$ since $\sum h_j\Delta\hat{F}_{KM} = 0$. Our second simplification uses the advanced time identity (see below) to rewrite the covariance expressions. We use the identity $n+1$ times for either the Kaplan–Meier CDF or the conditional Kaplan–Meier CDF to get

$$b_{jk} = \sum_{i=1}^{n}[h_j(T_i)-\bar{h}_j(T_i)][h_k(T_i)-\bar{h}_k(T_i)]\Delta\hat{F}_{KM}(T_i)$$

$$-\sum_{i=1}^{n}\frac{1-\delta_i}{n}\frac{\displaystyle\sum_{m:T_m>T_i}[h_j(T_m)-\bar{h}_j(T_m)][h_k(T_m)-\bar{h}_k(T_m)]\Delta\hat{F}_{KM}(T_m)}{1-\hat{F}_{KM}(T_i)}.$$

The third simplification uses the self-consistency identity again (with $g = [h_j - \bar{h}_j][h_k - \bar{h}_k]$). This allows us to combine the two terms. We get

$$b_{jk} = \sum_{i=1}^{n}[h_j(T_i)-\bar{h}_j(T_i)][h_k(T_i)-\bar{h}_k(T_i)]\frac{\delta_i}{n}.$$

The fourth and final simplification uses the following identity to replace δ_i/n:

$$\frac{\delta_i}{n(1-\hat{G}_{KM}(T_i))} = \Delta\hat{F}_{KM}(T_i).$$

ILLUSTRATION 73

This identity can be proved from the well-known fact for the Kaplan–Meier estimator $[1 - \hat{F}_{KM}(t)][1 - \hat{G}_{KM}(t)] = 1 - H(t)$.

Finally, the desired expression is as follows:

$$b_{jk} = \sum_{i=1}^{n} [h_j(T_i) - \bar{h}_j(T_i)][h_k(T_i) - \bar{h}_k(T_i)][1 - \hat{G}_{KM}(T_i)]\Delta\hat{F}_{KM}(T_i) .$$

Lemma 26 (*Advanced-time identity. Efron and Johnstone*) *Let us define the advanced time transformation for a function $g(t)$ with respect to a CDF $F(\cdot)$ as*

$$\bar{g}(s) = \bar{g}_F(s) = \frac{\int_{(s,\infty)} g(x)dF(x)}{1 - F(s)} = E_F[g(X)|X > s] .$$

Then we have

$$Var_F(g) = \int [g(x) - E_F g]^2 dF(x) = \int [g(x) - \bar{g}(x)]^2 dF(x)$$

and

$$Cov_F(g,h) = \int [g(t) - E_F g]h(t)dF(t) = \int [g(t) - \bar{g}(t)][h(t) - \bar{h}(t)]dF(t)$$

where $E_F g = \int g(x)dF(x)$.

PROOF: The result for the variance is directly from Efron and Johnstone [24]. The result for the covariance can be proved similarly. □

Lemma 27 (*Self-consistency identity*) *For the Kaplan–Meier estimator, $\hat{F}_{KM}$, we have that for any function $g(\cdot)$*

$$\sum_i g(T_i)\Delta\hat{F}_{KM}(T_i) = \sum_i \frac{\delta_i}{n}g(T_i) + \sum_i \frac{(1-\delta_i)}{n} \frac{\sum_{T_j > T_i} g(T_j)\Delta\hat{F}_{KM}(T_j)}{1 - \hat{F}_{KM}(T_i)} .$$

PROOF: The probability corresponding to $g(T_k)$ on the left-hand side is $\Delta\hat{F}_{KM}(T_k)$. The probabilities associated with $g(T_k)$ on the right-hand side are precisely those given by the Turnbull [118] self-consistent equation. It is well-known that the Kaplan–Meier estimator is self-consistent. □

3.3 Illustration

In survival analysis, the *median residual lifetime* at time x is defined as the median of the failure times conditional on the event that subjects survive beyond time x. Mathematically, suppose T is the survival time random variable under study. If $P(T - x > \theta | T > x) = 0.5$, then θ is the median of the remaining lifetimes at time x. Therefore, the median residual lifetime at x is quantitatively defined as the number θ that solves the equation

$$\frac{1 - F(x + \theta)}{1 - F(x)} = 0.5,$$

where $F(\cdot)$ is the cumulative distribution function of failure times. Other quantiles of the residual life distribution can be defined similarly. Even though we shall focus on developing the test for the median residual life function in what follows, the result can be easily modified to test any quantile residual life function.

Let us denote the median residual lifetime at time x as $Med(x)$. Clearly, $\theta = Med(x)$ is also the solution to

$$1 - F(x + \theta) = 0.5\{1 - F(x)\} .$$

After rearranging the terms, we see that θ is the solution to

$$0.5 = F(x + \theta) - 0.5F(x) .$$

If we define a function $g_b(t)$ as

$$g_b(t) = I[t \leq (x+b)] - 0.5I[t \leq x] - 0.5, \tag{3.17}$$

then the hypothesis $H_0 : Med(x) = b$ is equivalent to

$$H_0 : \int_0^\infty g_b(t)dF(t) = 0 .$$

This, in turn, can be accomplished by an empirical likelihood ratio test with a linear functional of the CDF.

We first determine the point estimator, taking $x = 365.25$ days.

```
data(cancer)
time <- cancer$time
status <- cancer$status-1
MMRtime(x=time, d=status, age=365.25)
## $MeanResidual
## [1] 275.9997
##
## $MedianResidual
## [1] 258.75
```

Next we code the g_b function defined in (3.17) as mygfun2( ) and then use el.cen.EM2( ) to test the hypothesis $H_0 : Med(365.25) = 300$.

```
mygfun2 <- function(s, age, Mdage){
    as.numeric(s<=(age+Mdage))-0.5*as.numeric(s<=age)-0.5}
el.cen.EM2(x=time, d=status, fun=mygfun2, mu=0,
                            age=365.25, Mdage=300)$Pval
## [1] 0.1192006
```

In order to find the confidence interval for $Med(365.25)$, we use the findUL( ) function.

ILLUSTRATION   75

```
myfunUL2 <- function(theta, x, d) {
            el.cen.EM2(x=x,d=d,fun=mygfun2,mu=0,
                       age=365.25,Mdage=theta) }
findUL(step=15, fun=myfunUL2, MLE=258, x=time,
                            d=status, level=2.70)
## $Low
## [1] 184.75
##
## $Up
## [1] 321.75
##
## $FstepL
## [1] 1.5e-07
##
## $FstepU
## [1] 1.5e-07
##
## $Lvalue
## [1] 2.503693
##
## $Uvalue
## [1] 2.427793
```

This calculation shows that a 90% confidence interval (since we set level = 2.70) for the median residual time at $x = 365.25$ is $[184.75, 321.75]$. Note we do not get the exact Lvalue and Uvalue of 2.70, which implies we do not get exact p-values of 0.1 here, due to the discrete nature of the quantile function.

Some people have advocated a smoothed quantile empirical likelihood ratio test. One way of smoothing the residual median is to replace the indicator functions in (3.17) by a smoothed version.

Smoothed version of the median:

```
mygfun22 <- function(s, age, Mdage) {
            myfun7(s, theta=(age+Mdage), epi=1/20) -
            0.5*myfun7(s, theta=age, epi=1/20) - 0.5 }
myfun7 <- function(x, theta=0, epi) {
          if(epi <= 0) stop("epi must > 0")
          u <- (x-theta)/epi
          return( pmax(0, pmin(1-u, 1)) ) }
```

By replacing the mygfun2 by mygfun22 in the above definition of the function myfunUL, we get the exact p-value or likelihood ratio value desired. The final confidence intervals are practically the same. In the function mygfun22 the epi value controls the smoothing slope. A value of $epi < 1/n$ where $n =$ sample size is recommended.

In a similar manner the mean residual lifetime of a survival random variable T, at a given time x, is defined as

$$M(x) = E(T|T \geq x) - x = \frac{\int_x^\infty s dF(s)}{1 - F(x)} - x = \frac{\int_x^\infty 1 - F(s) ds}{1 - F(x)}.$$

For a given x value, we first notice that the hypothesis

$$H_0: \quad M(x) = \mu$$

is equivalent to the hypothesis

$$H_0: \quad \frac{\int_x^\infty s dF(s)}{1 - F(x)} = (x + \mu) ,$$

which is also equivalent to

$$H_0: \quad \int_x^\infty s dF(s) = [1 - F(x)](x + \mu) .$$

This, in turn, can be written as (since $\int_x^\infty dF(s) = 1 - F(x)$)

$$H_0: \quad \int_x^\infty [s - (x + \mu)] dF(s) = 0 . \tag{3.18}$$

The above hypothesis can be tested by a one-sample empirical likelihood ratio test for censored survival data, similar to the median case, but with a different definition of the linear g function, i.e., $g(s) = [s - (x + \mu)] I[s > x]$.

```
mygfun <- function(s, age, muage) {
              as.numeric(s >= age)*(s-(age+muage))}
myfunUL <- function(theta, x, d) {
        el.cen.EM2(x=x, d=d, fun=mygfun,
                    mu=0, age=365.25, muage=theta)
}
findUL(step=15, fun=myfunUL, MLE=258, x=time,
                            d=status, level=2.70)
## $Low
## [1] 234.5338
##
## $Up
## [1] 323.1485
##
## $FstepL
## [1] 1.5e-07
##
## $FstepU
## [1] 1.5e-07
##
```

ILLUSTRATION 77

```
## $Lvalue
## [1] 2.7
##
## $Uvalue
## [1] 2.7
```

Therefore, the 90% confidence interval for the mean residual time at $x = 365.25$ days is $[234.53, 323.15]$.

Remark: We would like to point out that the variance of the median residual time or mean residual time with censored data is very difficult to estimate; thus a Wald-type confidence interval here is very impractical. We obtained the Wilks confidence interval without the variance estimator, which is another advantage of the empirical likelihood test.

Testing the equality (or the ratio) of two median residual times from two samples (or from one sample at two different times) can be carried out similarly as outlined in Jeong et al. [46].

For example, to test $H_0 : Med_1(x_1)/Med_2(x_2) = c$, where $Med_k(x_k)$ $(k = 1, 2)$ denotes the median residual time from sample k at time x_k, we would first obtain two empirical likelihood ratio statistics for testing two auxiliary hypotheses: $H_{01} : Med_1(x_1) = c\theta$ and $H_{02} : Med_2(x_2) = \theta$. Let us denote the two resulting test statistics by $W_1(c\theta; x_1)$ and $W_2(\theta; x_2)$. Then the original hypothesis $H_0 : Med_1(x_1)/Med_2(x_2) = c$ can be tested by using the statistic $W = \inf_\theta\{W_1(c\theta; x_1) + W_2(\theta; x_2)\}$, which follows a chi square distribution with 1 degree of freedom under H_0.

Specifically, to evaluate the test statistic under the null hypothesis of equality of two median residual lifetimes at a fixed time point (t_0), first fix c as 1 in the above H_0. Then for all possible support values of θ (recall that θ is also a time point), evaluate $W_k(\theta; t_0)$ in each group using the R function el.cen.EM2, denoting them as $W_1(\theta; t_0)$ and $W_2(\theta; t_0)$, respectively. Our observed two sample statistic is the minimum of the function $W = W_1(\theta; t_0) + W_2(\theta; t_0)$ over θ. Since W follows a χ^2 distribution with 1 degree of freedom (Jeong et al. [46]), the p-value associated with the observed value of the test statistic can be obtained using the chi square distribution.

Another special case is testing the ratio of two median residual lifetimes from the *same sample* but at two different times x_1 and x_2, i.e., $H_0 : Med(x_1)/Med(x_2) = c$. The inference procedure is similar to the above, except we replace the two auxiliary hypotheses by $H_{00} : Med(x_1) = c\theta$, $Med(x_2) = \theta$. Denote the test statistic as $W(c\theta, x_1; \theta, x_2)$. Finally, our test statistic for $H_0 : Med(x_1)/Med(x_2) = c$ is $\inf_\theta W(c\theta, x_1; \theta, x_2)$.

In addition to not requiring a nonparametric estimation of the density function for the variance calculation, the empirical likelihood ratio inference inherits the nice properties of a likelihood ratio based confidence region, i.e., range respecting and transform invariant.

3.4   Two Independent Samples

Suppose now that we have two independent samples of right censored survival data. We discuss here a class of two-sample empirical likelihood problems for which the parameter of interest can be written in the form

$$h(\theta_1, \theta_2) \tag{3.19}$$

for some R^2 to R^1 function $h(\cdot)$, where θ_1 is a parameter *only* of population 1 and θ_2 is a parameter *only* of population 2.

Remark: For more complicated two-sample parameters, the method discussed here will not work. For example, with parameters of the form

$$\theta = \int\int h(x, y)dF(x)dF(y)$$

please see the R package emplik2 and references therein for this type of two-sample problem.

Due to their independence, the empirical likelihood function for the two samples is simply the product of their empirical likelihoods; the log likelihood is the summation of their log empirical likelihoods. The maximum of the log empirical likelihood function for the two samples is achieved when each achieves its maximum, which are the two Kaplan–Meier estimators, as mentioned in Section 3.1.

To compute the empirical likelihood ratio, it is necessary to find the maximum of the two-sample empirical likelihood under the hypothesis $H_0 : h(\theta_1, \theta_2) = a$. Once we have that, the empirical likelihood ratio can be formed.

To this end, we assume the function h is such that, for any given constants a and b,

$$h(b, x) = a$$

always has a unique solution for x. Call this solution $h_b^{-1}a$. Then the computation of the empirical likelihood under $H_0 : h(\theta_1, \theta_2) = a$ can be accomplished in two steps. First, we compute the empirical likelihood under the hypothesis

$$H_{00} : \quad \theta_1 = b, \quad \theta_2 = h_b^{-1}a \ .$$

Let the resulting empirical likelihoods (from two samples) be called $W_1(b)$ and $W_2(b)$. The second step is to minimize $W_1(b) + W_2(b)$ over b. That is, $\inf_b(W_1(b) + W_2(b))$ is the desired empirical likelihood ratio under $H_0 : h(\theta_1, \theta_2) = a$.

Under the null hypothesis this likelihood ratio test will have a chi square distribution, following the approach of Naik-Nimbalkar and Rajarshi [76], who treated a k-sample median problem. We omit the details.

We next look at two examples where $h(\theta_1, \theta_2) = \theta_1 - \theta_2$ and $h(\theta_1, \theta_2) = \theta_1/\theta_2$, and leave other cases to the reader.

Example 15   *(Difference of two survival probabilities at a given time) The parameter of interest is*

$$D(t) = S_1(t) - S_2(t). \tag{3.20}$$

We first use empirical likelihood to test the hypothesis

$$H_0 : D(t) = a, \quad \text{for given } t \text{ and } a.$$

The key to our methodology is the following observation:

$$\max_{D(t)=a} \left(\log EL_1 + \log EL_2 \right) = \max_u \left(\max_{S_1(t)=u} \log EL_1 + \max_{S_2(t)=u-a} \log EL_2 \right),$$

where the two maximum values of $\log EL$ *in the right-hand side inside the parentheses are the same kind of constrained* $\log EL$ *that we computed for one-sample problems.*

Here is an R function for computing the empirical likelihood ratio to test (3.20). It requires the `emplik` *package.*

```
P1P2test <- function(theta, x1, d1, x2, d2,
                        t1=365.25, t2=365.25) {
a <- theta
Jointllr <- function(u, x1=x1, d1=d1, x2=x2, d2=d2, a=a) {
        temp1 <- el.cen.EM2(x=x1, d=d1,
    fun=function(x){as.numeric(x >= t1)}, mu = u)$"-2LLR"
    temp2 <- el.cen.EM2(x=x2, d=d2,
    fun=function(x){as.numeric(x >= t2)}, mu = u-a)$"-2LLR"
    return(temp1 + temp2)
  }
upBD <- min(0.999999, 1+a)
loBD <- max(0.000001, a)
temp <- optimize(f = Jointllr, lower = loBD, upper = upBD,
                x1 = x1, d1 = d1, x2 = x2, d2 = d2, a = a)
cstar <- temp$minimum
val <- temp$objective
pvalue <- 1 - pchisq( val, df=1)
tempMLE1 <- WKM(x=x1,d=d1)
tempMLE2 <- WKM(x=x2,d=d2)
P1 <- sum(tempMLE1$jump[(tempMLE1$times >= t1)])
P2 <- sum(tempMLE2$jump[(tempMLE2$times >= t2)])
MLE <- P1 - P2
list('-2LLR'=val, Dmle=MLE, ConstrMLE=cstar, Pval=pvalue)
}
```

Once we have defined the above function for testing the hypothesis (3.19), we can invert the test to obtain the confidence interval for the $D(t)$:

```
findUL(step=0.1, fun=P1P2test, MLE=0.24, x1=x1, d1=d1,
                                x2=x2, d2=d2)
```

Please note that the MLE for $D(t)$ *is part of the output from* `P1P2test`.

Example 16 *(Ratio of two failure probabilities) The parameter we are interested in is $F_1(t)/F_2(t)$. Again we first try to test the hypothesis*

$$H_0 : F_1(t)/F_2(t) = u \quad \text{for given } t \text{ and } u. \tag{3.21}$$

In the spirit of the previous example, we need an R function for calculating the two-sample log empirical likelihood function maximized under (3.21).

```
F1F2ratio <-
    function(theta, x1, d1, x2, d2, t1=365.25, t2=365.25) {
    a <- theta
Jointllr <- function(u, x1=x1, d1=d1, x2=x2, d2=d2, a=a) {
    temp1 <- el.cen.EM2(x=x1, d=d1,
        fun=function(x){as.numeric(x <= t1)}, mu = u)$"-2LLR"
    temp2 <- el.cen.EM2(x=x2, d=d2,
        fun=function(x){as.numeric(x <= t2)}, mu=u/a)$"-2LLR"
    return(temp1 + temp2)
                }
upBD <- min(0.999999, a)
loBD <- max(0.000001)
temp <- optimize(f = Jointllr, lower = loBD, upper = upBD,
                    x1 = x1, d1 = d1, x2 = x2, d2 = d2, a = a)
cstar <- temp$minimum
val <- temp$objective
pvalue <- 1 - pchisq(val, df=1)
tempMLE1 <- WKM(x=x1,d=d1)
tempMLE2 <- WKM(x=x2,d=d2)
P1 <- sum(tempMLE1$jump[(tempMLE1$times <= t1)])
P2 <- sum(tempMLE2$jump[(tempMLE2$times <= t2)])
MLE <- P1/P2
list('-2LLR'=val, Rmle=MLE, ConstrainMLE=cstar, Pval=pvalue)
}
```

Finally, the above test can be inverted (on u in 3.21) to obtain the confidence interval for the ratio of two failure probabilities at given time t:

```
findUL(step=0.1, fun=F1F2ratio, MLE=0.4187, x1=x1, d1=d1,
                                         x2=x2, d2=d2)
```

Recall that the confidence interval obtained this way has the *invariance property*: if we switch samples one and two, the MLE of the failure probability ratio is the reciprocal of the original ratio, and the confidence interval (upper and lower bounds) is also the reciprocal of the original confidence interval. Wald confidence intervals do not have this invariance property.

Remark: If we want to construct the Wald confidence interval for the difference $D(t)$, it is not clear what transformation we should apply, since the usual log transformation does not apply here, due to the possible negative value of $D(t)$. A similar difficulty occurs with the ratio of the failure probabilities. On the other hand, by inverting the likelihood ratio test we have no such concern about the transformation, since confidence intervals constructed in this way are transformation invariant.

3.5 Equality of k Medians

Naik-Nimbalkar and Rajarshi [76] have developed a theory for an empirical likelihood test for the equality of k medians with right censored data. But their paper contains no examples and no software. We can use el.cen.EM2( ) to compute the empirical likelihood test, with a procedure similar to the two-sample case above. However, in the profile calculation, we cannot use the optimize( ) function because the k empirical likelihoods involved are piecewise constant functions, and thus the usual check of the (numerical) derivative often fails.

One interesting thing is the way they arrive at the final log likelihood ratio for testing the equality of k medians. They first introduce an intermediate parameter θ and test the hypothesis that all k medians are equal to θ. This leads to a log likelihood ratio that has a chi square distribution with k degrees of freedom under the null hypothesis (that all k medians are actually θ). The final step is to profile out the intermediate parameter θ, by maximizing the log empirical likelihood ratio over all possible θ. In terms of the hypotheses, they first test the intermediate hypothesis

$$H_{00} : median_j = \theta, \quad \text{for } j = 1, 2, \cdots, k.$$

Upon profiling out θ, the null hypothesis becomes

$$H_0 : median_1 = \cdots = median_k .$$

We used this profiling procedure in the examples in Section 3.4 (for two samples) and we use it (for one sample) in Section 6.10 as well.

Theorem 28 *(Naik-Nimbalkar and Rajarshi) Suppose there are k independent samples. Assume each sample is generated from the random independent censorship model with lifetime distribution $F_i(t)$ and censoring distribution $G_i(t)$. Denote the sample sizes by n_i, $i = 1, 2, \cdots, k$.*

Assume $n_i/n \to \xi_i$, with $0 < \xi_i < 1$ when $n \to \infty$. Here $n = \sum_{i=1}^{k} n_i$.

Let $W_i(\theta)$ denote the -2 log empirical likelihood ratio for testing the median of sample i equal to θ. Define

$$W(\theta) = \sum_{i=1}^{k} W_i(\theta).$$

Finally, assume $F_i(t)$ $i = 1, 2, \cdots, k$ have a common median m and $F_i(t)$ is continuous in a neighborhood of the median with a positive density: $dF_i(x)/dx|_{x=m} = f_i(m) > 0$. Finally, assume $1 - G_i(m) > 0$.

Then, we have, as $n \to \infty$,

$$\inf_{\theta} W(\theta) \longrightarrow \chi^2_{k-1}$$

in distribution.

Furthermore, the infimum is achieved by one or more values of θ. If we denote the value of θ that achieves the infimum above by $\hat{\theta}$, then

$$\min_{1 \leq i \leq k} (\hat{\theta}_i) \leq \hat{\theta} \leq \max_{1 \leq i \leq k} (\hat{\theta}_i) \tag{3.22}$$

where $\hat{\theta}_i$ is the Kaplan–Meier median from sample i.

PROOF: See the paper by Naik-Nimbalkar and Rajarshi [76]. □

In the paper they also calculated the common median, $\hat{\theta}$, defined in (3.22), and it is a convex combination of the k Kaplan–Meier medians. This also offers an example of the "overdetermined" estimating equations, since we have k samples and each sample offers an estimator, the Kaplan–Meier median. Yet the common median $\hat{\theta}$ is better than any of the k medians based on individual samples. It pools the information from all k samples and combines them in an optimal way.

Example 17 *(Testing the equality of k medians) We use the dataset "larynx" in the package* `KMsurv` *to illustrate the computation. In this dataset, there is a variable "stage" and there are four different stages. We shall test the hypothesis that all four survival curves (corresponding to the four stages) have same median.*

Assume the survival times from four different stages are independent, we use the empirical likelihood test of Naik-Nimbalkar and Rajarshi, i.e., compute the p-value.

```
data(larynx)
larynx1 <- subset(larynx, stage == 1)
larynx2 <- subset(larynx, stage == 2)
larynx3 <- subset(larynx, stage == 3)
larynx4 <- subset(larynx, stage == 4)
JointLLR4 <- function(theta, data1, data2, data3, data4) {
      Medfun <- function(x){ as.numeric(x <= theta) - 0.5 }
      temp1 <- el.cen.EM2(x=data1$time, d=data1$delta,
                                      fun=Medfun, mu=0)
      temp2 <- el.cen.EM2(x=data2$time, d=data2$delta,
                                      fun=Medfun, mu=0)
      temp3 <- el.cen.EM2(x=data3$time, d=data3$delta,
                                      fun=Medfun, mu=0)
      temp4 <- el.cen.EM2(x=data4$time, d=data4$delta,
                                      fun=Medfun, mu=0)
return(temp1$"-2LLR" + temp2$"-2LLR"+
                            temp3$"-2LLR" + temp4$"-2LLR")
}
```

Now we need to minimize the $-2LLR$ over the `theta`, *the common value of the median. Since the empirical likelihood ratio for the median is not smooth (in fact, it is piecewise constant) we cannot use a standard minimum seeking algorithm. Fortunately, we only need to search between the four individual medians, and due to the*

*piecewise constant property of the EL, we only need to search one point in between
every two consecutive observations there.*

*These four datasets have medians 6.5, 7, 5, 1.5, respectively. So we only need to
search within the interval* $(1.5, 7)$.

```
thetavec <- 1:100/20 + 1.5
for(i in 1:100)
    aa[i] <- JointLLR4(theta=thetavec[i], larynx1,
                             larynx2, larynx3, larynx4)
min(aa)
thetavec[which.min(aa)]
## [1] 4.05
JointLLR4(theta=4.05, larynx1, larynx2,larynx3,larynx4)
## [1] 15.36998

> 1-pchisq(15.36998, df=3)
## [1] 0.001526279
```

The values of $-2LLR$ *over 400 are uninteresting. We see the minimum of* $-2LLR$
is 15.36998, achieved when `theta` *is approximately 4.05 to 4.25*

The location of the minimum, $\theta = 4.15$, *is also the maximum empirical likelihood estimator of the common median. This is an example of an over-determined
estimating equation.*

The minimum value of $-2LLR$ *(=15.36998), corresponds to a p-value of
0.001526279. The degrees of freedom for the chi square distribution is equal to number of groups minus one, i.e.,* $4 - 1 = 3$.

*We see that the last group (with stage = 4, median = 1.5) is markedly different
from the other three groups. Perhaps a more interesting question is to test if the first
three groups, with stages = 1, 2 or 3, have the same medians. We shall not repeat
the code for function* `JointLLR3` *here since it is similar to the four group case. If we
test the equality of the medians for the first three groups, the p-value calculation is
as follows.*

The minimum is achieved when `theta` *= 6.2, and the* $-2LLR$ *is 1.11875*

```
thetavec <- 1:100/50 + 5.5
for(i in 1:100)
    aa[i] <- JointLLR3(theta=thetavec[i], larynx1,
                             larynx2, larynx3)
plot(thetavec, aa)
min(aa)
## [1] 1.11875
which.min(aa)
## [1] 35
thetavec[35]
## [1] 6.2
JointLLR3(theta=thetavec[35], larynx1, larynx2,larynx3)
```

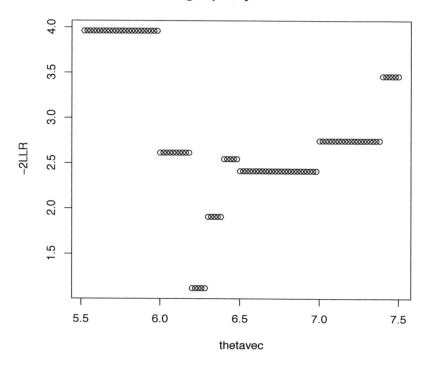

Figure 3.2: Minimizing over the piecewise constant -2 log empirical likelihood ratios.

```
## [1] 1.11875
1-pchisq(1.11875, df=2)
## [1] 0.5715662
```

We see the test of equal median among the first three groups has p-value 0.5715662. The maximum empirical likelihood estimator of the common median of the first three groups is 6.2, see Fig. 3.2.

The confidence interval of the common median for the first three groups can also be obtained by inverting the test. We leave this to the reader.

3.6   Functionals of the CDF and Functionals of Hazard

This section can be omitted in the first reading and will not interrupt the flow of the rest of the material. In this section we first discuss the topic of approximating $\int g(t)d(F(t) - F_0(t))$ by the hazard counterpart $\int \tilde{g}(t)d(\Lambda(t) - \Lambda_0(t))$. This relation connects the results of Chapter 2 to those of Chapter 3. The representation we obtained leads to another proof of the Wilks theorem for empirical likelihood ratio testing for the estimating equations in terms of the CDF.

We begin with a lemma. See Gill [35] for a proof.

Lemma 29 *Suppose $F_1(t)$ and $F_2(t)$ are two arbitrary distribution functions. The corresponding cumulative hazard functions are denoted by $\Lambda_1(t)$ and $\Lambda_2(t)$. We have the identity*

$$\frac{F_1(t) - F_2(t)}{1 - F_2(t)} = \int_{-\infty}^{t} \frac{1 - F_1(s-)}{1 - F_2(s)} d[\Lambda_1(s) - \Lambda_2(s)] , \qquad (3.23)$$

provided $1 - F_2(t) > 0$.

This is a well-known result (Duhamel's equation); see, for example, Gill [35]. When $F_2(t)$ is taken to be the "true" CDF and $F_1(t)$ to be the Kaplan–Meier estimator (thus $\Lambda_1(t)$ is the Nelson–Aalen estimator), this lemma has been used by many other authors in various places, for example, Gill [36]. Our desire is to point out that this result is true for *any* pair of CDFs, and we shall use it for estimators other than the Kaplan–Meier/Nelson–Aalen pair.

Lemma 30 *Suppose $F_1(t)$ and $F_2(t)$ are two arbitrary distribution functions. The corresponding cumulative hazard functions are denoted by $\Lambda_1(t)$ and $\Lambda_2(t)$. Suppose $\phi(t)$ is an integrable function. Then we have*

$$\int_{-\infty}^{\infty} \phi(t) d[F_1(t) - F_2(t)] \qquad (3.24)$$

$$= \int_{\infty}^{\infty} \left\{ [1 - F_1(t-)][\phi(t) - \frac{\int_t^{\infty} \phi(u) dF_2(u)}{1 - F_2(t)}] \right\} d[\Lambda_1(t) - \Lambda_2(t)] .$$

In the above identity, if we take $F_2(t)$ to be the "true" CDF $F_0(t)$ and $F_1(t)$ to be the Kaplan–Meier estimator (thus $\Lambda_1(t)$ is the Nelson–Aalen estimator), then the identity above is related to the so-called i.i.d. representation of the Kaplan–Meier integral, since the integration of hazard is very nearly a sum of i.i.d. terms:

$$\int \tilde{g}(t) d(\hat{\Lambda}_{NA}(t) - \Lambda_0(t)) = \frac{1}{n} \sum_{i=1}^{n} \frac{\tilde{g}(T_i)\delta_i}{1 - \hat{H}(T_i)} - \int \tilde{g}(t) d\Lambda_0(t)$$

where $1 - \hat{H}(t) = R(t)/n$. If we replace $1 - \hat{H}(t)$ in the above by its limit $1 - H(t)$, then the right-hand side may be viewed as an i.i.d. representation, i.e., the following is a sum with terms that are i.i.d. with mean zero:

$$\frac{1}{n} \sum_{i=1}^{n} \frac{\tilde{g}(T_i)\delta_i}{1 - H(T_i-)} - \int \tilde{g}(t) d\Lambda_0(t) .$$

Akritas [2] studied such approximations and explicitly computed $\tilde{g}(t)$. He showed that the approximation has error $o_p(1/\sqrt{n})$ and then used it in a proof of the CLT for the Kaplan–Meier integral.

We would, however, allow $F_1(t)$ to be *any* CDF that is dominated by the Kaplan–Meier estimator and is within an $O(1/\sqrt{n})$ neighborhood of the Kaplan–Meier estimator. On the other hand, if we allow the weight function $\tilde{g}(t)$ to be predictable, by the martingale central limit theorem we can easily manage the predictable integrand. The following lemma gives the function $\tilde{g}(t)$ explicitly and concludes that the error of the approximation is $o(1/\sqrt{n})$.

Let $\tau_n = \max_i T_i$. Without loss of generality, we assume $\tau_n \to \infty$ as $n \to \infty$.

First, we point out that a key relationship (also used by Akritas) holds not only when $\hat{F}$ and $\hat{\Lambda}$ are the Kaplan–Meier/Nelson–Aalen pair, but also for *any* CDF/cumulative hazard pair:

$$\int_{-\infty}^{\tau_n} g(t) d(\hat{F}(t) - F_0(t)) = \int_{-\infty}^{\tau_n} \tilde{g}(t) d(\hat{\Lambda}(t) - \Lambda_0(t)). \qquad (3.25)$$

The identity (3.25) is derived from identity (3.23) or (3.24). The weight function in (3.25) is

$$\tilde{g}(t) = (1 - \hat{F}(t-)) \left[g(t) - \frac{\int_t^{\tau_n} g(u) dF_0(u)}{1 - F_0(t)} \right]. \qquad (3.26)$$

Then, following the same analysis in Akritas [2], we replace τ_n by ∞ in the definition of $\tilde{g}(t)$ (calling it $g^*(t)$), and the above equality (3.25) becomes an approximation with error rate $o_p(1/\sqrt{n})$.

As discussed before, we may restrict our attention to those CDFs and hazard functions that are dominated by the Kaplan–Meier/Nelson–Aalen estimator and are in a $O(1/\sqrt{n})$ neighborhood (in sup norm) of the Kaplan–Meier/Nelson–Aalen estimator.

Lemma 31 *Given an i.i.d. right censored sample (T_i, δ_i). Suppose $F(t)$ is a CDF and $\Lambda(t)$ is the corresponding cumulative hazard function. We restrict our attention to those $F(t)$ or those $\Lambda(t)$ that are dominated by the Kaplan–Meier or Nelson–Aalen estimator. Furthermore, we assume $\Lambda(t)$ are within $O(1/\sqrt{n})$ of the Nelson–Aalen estimator, i.e., for any $0 < \tau < \infty$*

$$\sup_{t \le \tau} |\Lambda(t) - \hat{\Lambda}_{NA}(t)| = O_p(1/\sqrt{n}) .$$

We suppose also that

$$\int_{-\infty}^{\infty} \frac{g(t)}{1 - G(t-)} dF(t) < \infty ,$$

where the function $G(\cdot)$ is the CDF of the censoring variable. Then

$$\int_{-\infty}^{\infty} g(t) d(F(t) - F_0(t)) = \int_{-\infty}^{\infty} g^*(t) d(\Lambda(t) - \Lambda_0(t)) + o_p(1/\sqrt{n}) ,$$

where $F_0(t)$ and $\Lambda_0(t)$ are the true CDF and cumulative hazard, respectively. The definition of $g^*(t)$ is almost the same as (3.26) except τ is replaced by ∞ there.

3.6.1   Alternative Proof of the Wilks Theorem for Means

Here we present an alternative proof of the Wilks theorem for mean functions, i.e., Theorem 23. This proof is perhaps a more elegant approach to the proof of the Wilks theorem for linear functionals of a CDF. It makes use of the results for the hazard linear functionals in Chapter 2.

Simply put, this approach attempts to approximate and replace the constraint or hypothesis, formulated in terms of the CDF, by the constraint in terms of linear functionals of the hazard.

The idea of approximating mean functions of the Kaplan–Meier estimator by functionals of the Nelson–Aalen estimator has been used by other authors. In particular, the so-called i.i.d. representation of the Kaplan–Meier estimator falls into this category. The most relevant paper to our discussion here is Akritas [2].

Note that $\tilde{g}(t)$ in Lemma 31 above is predictable and converges to g^*.

(1) We need to verify that the approximation in Lemma 31 has an error of $o_p(1/\sqrt{n})$. This is similar to the proof in Akritas [2].

(2) The approximation is not only valid for the Kaplan–Meier and Nelson–Aalen pair, but is also valid for any CDF/hazard pair in an $O(1/\sqrt{n})$ neighborhood of the Kaplan–Meier or Nelson–Aalen estimator.

In view of the lemma, we may replace the empirical likelihood with constraints of CDF linear functionals by the empirical likelihood with constraints of hazard linear functionals. In other words, the hypothesis

$$H_0 : \int g(t)d(F(t) - F_0(t)) = 0$$

is equivalent to the hypothesis

$$H_0 : \int \tilde{g}(t)d(\Lambda(t) - \Lambda_0(t)) = o_p(1/\sqrt{n}) \ .$$

The EL analysis for the latter hypothesis has been treated in Chapter 2; thus we obtain the Wilks theorem of the CDFs.

The fact that $\tilde{g}(t)$ involves $F_0(t)$ should not cause any alarm.

3.7   Predictable Mean Function

Using the hazard functional approximation for the mean functional, it is easy to generalize the empirical likelihood ratio Wilks theorem (Theorem 23) to include the case where the mean functions are defined by integrands that are random but "predictable."

We only state the result here. This theorem is useful for the analysis of the Buckley–James estimator in Chapter 5.

Theorem 32 *In the context of Theorem 23, suppose we are testing for the hypothesis*

$$H_0 : \int g_{nr}(t)dF(t) = 0; \quad r = 1, 2, \cdots, p. \tag{3.27}$$

where $g_{nr}(t)$ are random but "predictable" functions.

Assume (i) For any given τ such that $F_0(\tau) < 1$, we have $\sup_{t \leq \tau} |g_{nr}(t) - g_r(t)| \to$ 0 in probability as $n \to \infty$. The limit functions $g_r(t)$ are nonrandom functions that satisfy the requirements of Theorem 23.

(ii) As $n \to \infty$, the following ratios are bounded in probability:

$$\sup_i \frac{g_{nr}(T_i)}{g_r(T_i)} \ .$$

Then the conclusions of Theorem 23 are still valid for testing the hypothesis (3.27). In particular, the -2 log likelihood ratio under the null hypothesis (3.27) has asymptotically a chi square distribution with degrees of freedom p.

3.8   Discussion, Historic Notes, and Remarks

For right censored data, Thomas and Grunkemeier [112] proposed using empirical likelihood as a way of constructing a confidence interval for a single parameter of survival probability at a fixed time point. They compared this method with competing methods and showed its advantages. This is the first time that empirical likelihood was proposed as a better nonparametric inference method. Li [67] and Murphy [74] made the arguments in Thomas and Grunkemeier (1975) rigorous.

For a single parameter of mean integral, and *doubly censored* data, Murphy and van der Vaart [75] demonstrated an asymptotic chi square distribution for the empirical likelihood ratio. But the conditions imposed, like boundedness of integrand and bounded support, were often too restrictive in practice.

The empirical likelihood test for the equality of k medians from k independent samples was studied by Naik-Nimbalkar and Rajarshi [76]. They showed that the empirical likelihood ratio test statistic under the null hypothesis has a chi square distribution with $k-1$ degrees of freedom. This apparently is the first empirical likelihood Wilks theorem in survival analysis that yields a chi square limit with $k > 1$ degrees of freedom.

Pan [83] and Pan and Zhou [84] studied the empirical likelihood ratio tests for hazard functionals.

Owen's book [81] contains some results on the censored data empirical likelihood ratio test. Although many special cases have appeared before, Theorem 23 seems new, in that it deals with k constraints and allows the constraints to be formulated in general linear functionals of CDF.

The advantage of empirical likelihood confidence intervals is inherited from the parametric counterpart and is discussed by DiCiccio et al. [21].

On the other hand, there are many papers in the literature dealing with *pseudo* empirical likelihood tests for right censored data with parameters defined by multiple mean functions. These methods do not modify the likelihood of Owen for i.i.d. samples and are simpler algebraically to manipulate. However, pseudo empirical likelihood can be sub-optimal in many cases. See the many examples in Hjort et al. [40]. See also our discussion in Chapter 7 for the comparison of the size and the shape of the confidence regions derived from various empirical likelihood ratio tests.

In the analysis of (multiple) linear regression models, the least-squares type methods lead to the so-called normal equations. If the linear model has p covariates, then we end up with $p+1$ simultaneous estimating equations. To apply EL techniques, we need a Wilks theorem with multiple $(p+1)$ parameters. Thus our result in this chapter is needed in the EL analysis of censored data regression models (AFT models), where typically multiple estimating equations of mean type, with terms that are not necessarily bounded, are involved (see Chapter 5).

Another example where the Wilks theorem for EL is useful is in the testing of mean residual lifetimes (Zhou and Jeong [140]), where the terms are again not bounded and estimation of the standard error of the NPMLE is difficult.

3.9   Exercises

Exercise 3.1 *By inverting the empirical likelihood ratio test, find the 90% confidence interval of the common median in the context of Example 17.*

Exercise 3.2 *Similar to Example 16, use the same data there to test the hypothesis that $H_0 : S_1(365.25)/S_2(365.25) = 1$, where $S_i(t) = 1 - F_i(t)$.*

Chapter 4

Empirical Likelihood Analysis of the Cox Model

In this chapter we discuss two different empirical likelihood schemes for the Cox proportional hazards regression model. The first approach is to construct the empirical likelihood on the observed data, assuming it comes from a Cox model. The second approach, which we only discuss briefly, is to construct the EL based on the estimating equations given by Cox. Differences and similarities to the Cox partial likelihood are discussed. Joint inference involving the baseline hazard and regression parameters are studied. We also illustrate how the empirical likelihood method can be applied to an extension of the proportional hazards model proposed by Yang and Prentice [129].

4.1 Introduction

The most widely used regression model in survival analysis is the Cox proportional hazards model, introduced by Cox in [15] and [16]. It is a regression model formulated in terms of hazard functions rather than distribution functions or means. It is similar to the exponential regression model but without the exponential distribution assumption.

The Cox model includes the log rank test as the score test and the Nelson–Aalen estimator (and thus the Kaplan–Meier estimator) as the baseline hazard estimator, so it encompasses the two most important topics in survival analysis. The study of the Cox model has stimulated many new developments in statistics and probability. For example, the theory and application of counting processes and martingales became a hot topic after the Cox model connection, and it is now part of the standard toolbox in survival analysis. The Cox proportional hazards regression model is also the starting point of many extensions. We include one such extension in Section 4.5.

Let $X_1, \cdots, X_n$ be nonnegative independent random variables, denoting lifetimes, and $z_1, \cdots, z_n$ be the covariates associated with survival times $X_1, \cdots, X_n$. In this section we assume z_i do not change with time (i.e., not time-change covariates). In practice, the covariates z_i might represent the gender, age and treatment information of the ith patient.

The Cox proportional hazards regression model stipulates that the *hazard func-*

tion, $\lambda_i(t)$, of the ith lifetime X_i, is related to the covariate z_i in the following fashion:

$$\lambda_{X_i}(t) = \lambda_i(t) = \lambda(t|z_i) = \lambda_0(t)\exp(\beta_0 z_i) , \qquad (4.1)$$

where β_0 is an unknown regression coefficient and $\lambda_0(t)$ is the so-called baseline hazard function. Another way to think of $\lambda_0(t)$ is that it is the hazard function for an individual with zero covariates, $z = 0$.

There are two unknown components in the Cox model: the baseline hazard function $\lambda_0(t)$ and the regression coefficient β_0. The Cox proportional hazards model assumes that the baseline hazard function $\lambda_0(t)$ is a completely unknown and arbitrary function (nonparametric), but is common to all patients; and the regression coefficient β_0 is a finite dimensional parameter. If z and β_0 have dimension > 1, then $\beta_0 z_i$ above should be understood as the inner product. Such nonparametric/parametric mixed models are often called semi-parametric models.

The key feature in the model is the assumption that the ratio of any two hazard functions is a constant and does not depend on time t, thus the name "proportional hazards." That the constant ratio be exponential in $\beta_0 z$ is not critical. The exponential function happens to be a function that is always positive and easy to work with when we take the log of the likelihood.

Arbitrary baseline but constant hazard ratio strikes a nice balance between the tractability and flexibility of the model, making Cox proportional hazards model the first choice in survival regression modeling.

Another way to think of the Cox proportional hazards model is that it is an exponential regression model but the responses have undergone an arbitrary, crazy clock time change; see Zhou [136].

Finally, the lifetimes X_i are subject to right censoring; therefore, what we actually observe is not X_i, z_i but

$$T_i = \min(X_i, C_i), \quad \delta_i = I[X_i \leq C_i] \quad \text{and} \quad z_i \qquad (4.2)$$

where C_i are censoring times, assumed to be independent of X_i given the z_i.

Cox in [15] and [16] not only proposed the model, he actually gave us the so-called *partial likelihood function*, making the analysis of the model tractable. Since then, the model and partial likelihood have been well studied. Many of those results are now included in survival analysis textbooks like Kalbfleisch and Prentice [51] and Therneau and Grambsch [111]. Fleming and Harrington [28] or Andersen et al. [3] contain more advanced materials focused on counting process martingale theory.

We include a theorem about the asymptotic property of the Cox maximum partial likelihood estimator due to Andersen and Gill [4] without proof at the end of this chapter.

4.2   Empirical Likelihood Analysis of the Cox Model

We begin with the definition of the empirical likelihood function for data coming from a Cox model. Since the Cox model is formulated in terms of hazard, it is more convenient to use empirical likelihood in terms of hazard. It turns out that the Poisson version of the hazard likelihood (see Chapter 1) is the easiest to work with.

Remark: Due to the continuous/discrete issues of the hazard function, slightly different versions of the empirical likelihood can be formulated for the Cox model. See Ren and Zhou [96]. The difference may be significant in the case of small sample size, or when underlying survival distributions are discrete. However, assuming continuous lifetime distributions, these differences will vanish as sample size increases. We will not discuss it further here but refer the interested readers to Ren and Zhou [96].

The contribution to the (Poisson version of) empirical likelihood function from a single right censored observation (T_i, δ_i) is (see 1.27)

$$\{\lambda_i(T_i)dt_i\}^{\delta_i} \exp\{-\Lambda_i(T_i)\}. \tag{4.3}$$

Under Cox's proportional hazards model, we have

$$\lambda_i(T_i) = \lambda_0(T_i)\exp(\beta z_i), \quad \text{and} \quad \Lambda_i(T_i) = \Lambda_0(T_i)\exp(\beta z_i).$$

Also, assuming a purely discrete cumulative hazard that has possible jumps only at the observed survival times, T_i (see below for explanation of this assumption), we can write

$$\lambda_0(T_i)dt_i = \Delta\Lambda_0(T_i) \quad \text{and} \quad \Lambda_0(T_i) = \sum_{j:T_j \leq T_i} \Delta\Lambda_0(T_j) \,.$$

By substituting these into (4.3) above, and aggregating all n observations, the empirical likelihood function for all n right censored observations under Cox's model is

$$Lik_{emp} = \mathcal{AL}^c(\beta, \Lambda_0) = \prod_{i=1}^{n}(\Delta\Lambda_0(T_i)e^{\beta z_i})^{\delta_i}\exp\{-e^{\beta z_i}\sum_{j:T_j \leq T_i} \Delta\Lambda_0(T_j)\} \,. \tag{4.4}$$

Although the baseline hazard is arbitrary, when maximizing the empirical likelihood with respect to the baseline, we shall restrict ourselves to those hazard functions that are dominated by $\hat{\Lambda}_{NA}$, the Nelson–Aalen estimator based on the data $(T_i, \delta_i), i = 1, 2, \ldots, n$. That is, we seek to maximize the empirical likelihood only over those discrete hazard functions that have the same jump points as the Nelson–Aalen estimator, or jumps only at observed event times. This restriction is similar to that of $F \ll \hat{F}_n$ for CDFs imposed by Owen [78] when he seeks to maximize the empirical likelihood in terms of distribution functions. Basically, Owen showed that some restriction is necessary and this particular restriction is a reasonable one. See Owen [78] for more discussion. See also Li [67] for some related discussion. Intuitively, the maximization forces the candidates CDF to be discrete and jump only at the observed times. There is no restriction on the β value when we do the maximization.

We discuss below two approaches when maximizing the empirical likelihood (4.4). First, if our focus is on the regression parameter β alone, then we can "profile out" the baseline, i.e., maximize the (log) empirical likelihood with respect to the baseline for fixed (but arbitrary) β, and this leads to a log likelihood that depends only on β. We shall see that this is the same (besides a constant) as the well-known Cox log partial likelihood. Second, if our interest is in both β *and* the baseline hazard (for example, the survival of a patient with a particular covariate), we shall work directly with the empirical likelihood above, simultaneously maximizing over β and the baseline hazard.

For easy comparison, we also list here the log "partial likelihood" of Cox; see, for example, the book by Kalbfleisch and Prentice [51]. Notice that the Cox partial likelihood is a function of β only while empirical likelihood is a function of both β and the baseline hazard function.

Log Cox partial likelihood:

$$\log Lik_{cox}(\beta) = \sum_{i=1}^{n} \delta_i \left(\beta z_i - \log \left[\sum_j e^{\beta z_j} I[t_j \geq t_i] \right] \right). \tag{4.5}$$

The log of the empirical likelihood function (4.4) above, with $w_i = \Delta \Lambda_0(T_i)$:

$$\log Lik_{emp}(\beta, w_i) = \sum_{i=1}^{n} \delta_i(\beta z_i + \log w_i) - \sum_{i=1}^{n} \left(e^{\beta z_i} \sum_j w_j I[t_j \leq t_i] \right). \tag{4.6}$$

The $\log Lik_{emp}$ is obtained by taking the log of $\mathcal{AL}^c$ defined in (4.4).

When there are tied observations, several modifications to the Cox partial likelihood (4.5) are available. There is a whole section discussing various ways of handling tied data in the Cox model in Therneau and Grambsch's book [111]. Similar modifications are possible for EL. For simplicity, we consider only data with no ties below.

4.2.1   Profile out the Baseline

We look at the approach of profiling out the baseline in more detail now.

Assume for the moment that β is fixed and we shall maximize the $\log Lik_{emp}$ over w_i's. It is not hard to calculate (taking the derivative and setting the derivative to zero) that the value of w_j that maximize the $\log Lik_{emp}$, for any given β, is

$$w_i(\beta) = \frac{\delta_i}{\sum_j e^{\beta z_j} I[t_j \geq t_i]}. \tag{4.7}$$

If we plug the expression for $w_i(\beta)$ back into the log empirical likelihood (4.6) and switch the order of the two summations in the second term on the right-hand side, we can compute

$$\log Lik_{emp} = \log Lik_{cox} - \sum_j \delta_j .$$

We put this fact into a formal theorem:

Theorem 33 *Assume there are no ties in the observed event times. The log partial likelihood of Cox (4.5) and the log empirical likelihood (4.6), after profiling out the baseline, are almost the same. The difference is equal to the number of uncensored observations in the sample.*

Proof: Use the definition of the two log likelihoods (4.5) and (4.6) and the calculation is straightforward. □

Remark: Since the number of uncensored observations does not involve the regression parameter β, the (nonparametric) maximum likelihood estimators from the two likelihoods will always be the same. The likelihood ratio will also be the same whether we use partial likelihood or profiled empirical likelihood.

Definition: *We denote the maximum partial likelihood estimator of the regression parameter as $\hat{\beta}_c$. In view of the above remark, this is also the NPMLE, the estimator that maximizes the empirical likelihood of (4.6).*

We shall also call the baseline estimator, $w_i(\hat{\beta}_c)$, the Breslow estimator; it is (4.7) with $\beta = \hat{\beta}_c$.

Remark: the relation between the two log likelihoods only holds when there is no constraint on the baseline. Obviously, there is no such relation when there is a constraint on the baseline, since the Cox partial likelihood does not involve the baseline hazard, and thus affords no place for a constraint on the baseline.

The immediate consequence of Theorem 33 and the following is formulated in the theorem below:

Theorem 34 *(Pan [83]) Under the same regularity conditions that guarantee the asymptotic normality of the Cox partial likelihood estimator (see Section 4.7), we have*

$$-2\log \frac{\sup_{\{\Lambda_0\}} \mathcal{AL}^c(\beta_0, \Lambda_0)}{\sup_{\{\beta, \Lambda_0\}} \mathcal{AL}^c(\beta, \Lambda_0)} = (\beta_0 - \hat{\beta}_c)I(\xi)(\beta_0 - \hat{\beta}_c)^{\top}, \qquad (4.8)$$

where ξ lies between β_0 and $\hat{\beta}_c$ and $I(\cdot)$ is the information matrix from the partial likelihood. See Section 4.7 for a full definition of $I(\cdot)$.

Consequently, as $n \to \infty$,

$$-2\log \frac{\sup_{\{\Lambda_0\}} \mathcal{AL}^c(\beta_0, \Lambda_0)}{\sup_{\{\beta, \Lambda_0\}} \mathcal{AL}^c(\beta, \Lambda_0)} \xrightarrow{\mathcal{D}} \chi^2_{(p)}. \qquad (4.9)$$

We recall that in the above expression the sup over Λ_0 is restricted to those Λ_0 that are dominated by the Nelson–Aalen estimator: $\Lambda_0 \ll \Lambda_{NA}$. The above results also imply that the (profile) empirical likelihood ratio test concerning β's is the same as the Cox partial likelihood ratio test. The latter is available in popular software packages (SAS, R, etc.). Therefore, no special software is needed for the empirical likelihood ratio test here.

4.2.2   Inference Involving Baseline

In the Cox model, the regression coefficient β determines only the *ratio* of two hazards, i.e., it tells the *relative* value of one hazard to another. If you want to find the hazard function itself or the survival probability itself, for example, as a prediction, you need both the baseline and the coefficient β. For example, the 5-year survival probability for a patient with covariate z, based on the Cox model, is $\exp(-\hat{\Lambda}_0(5)e^{\hat{\beta}_c z})$.

One could use the joint asymptotic normality of $\hat{\beta}_c$ and Breslow's baseline estimator and delta method to calculate the asymptotic variance of the parameters. See Tsiatis [116] for the calculation of the joint variance.

When the parameter of interest becomes more complicated (for example, in a stratified Cox proportional hazards model, etc.), the calculation of variance becomes more complicated. In addition, confidence intervals based on the asymptotic normality calculation often need to be coupled with a transformation in order to achieve good coverage probability in small to medium samples. But for more complicated cases, it is not clear what kind of transformation to use, and the computation of the variance estimators is burdensome.

An alternative approach is to use empirical likelihood for inferences involving both β and baseline hazard. The empirical likelihood ratio test can be computed without the asymptotic variance, and the related confidence interval does not require a parameter transformation. The test procedure is easy to perform with a computer. The confidence intervals can then be obtained by inverting the EL test. The inversion procedure is conceptually easy. But for problems with many parameters, the inversion calculations sometimes require a long computation time, since we must search for the maximum and minimum of a function with many variables over a (multidimensional) convex domain. However, we argue that this type of difficulty can be tackled by the vast modern computational power. See our examples in this chapter and Chapter 6 for further discussion.

The confidence interval based on empirical likelihood does not require transformation on the parameter. In fact, it is transformation invariant. Therefore, even if we apply a transformation, the resulting confidence interval will remain the same.[1] In this sense the confidence interval so obtained is like the interval where "the best transformation" has been applied.

We end this section with one more scenario in which we require joint inference for β and the baseline. For example, in the stratified proportional hazards model case, we might want to compare the cumulative hazards of two strata at a given time

---

[1] We mean the confidence interval for the original parameter θ, and for its transformation $h(\theta)$, will be $[A, B]$ and $[h(A), h(B)]$, assuming the function h is monotone increasing. Otherwise, the latter confidence interval will be $[\min h(\theta), \max h(\theta)]$ where the min and max are taken over $\theta \in [A, B]$.

point a: $\Lambda_0(a)$ vs. $\Lambda_1(a)$; by the Cox model this is estimated by $\hat{\Lambda}_0(a)$ and $e^{\hat{\beta}}\hat{\Lambda}_0(a)$. The difference of the two estimates is then $\hat{\Lambda}_0(a)[1 - e^{\hat{\beta}}]$. To determine whether the confidence interval of the difference includes zero, we require a joint confidence region of β and $\Lambda_0(a)$. The difference of hazards is also equivalent to the so-called survival probability ratio (after a log transformation).

Another case that involves joint inference is the stratified Cox model. Since unnecessary stratification reduces the power of tests, we may want to merge strata. In that case we will work with the ratio of the two baseline hazards from different strata at several given time points.

4.2.3 Parameters θ and λ

In this section we demonstrate how to use empirical likelihood to make a joint inference involving the Breslow baseline hazard estimator and the Cox partial likelihood estimator. First, we show how to test a hypothesis that involves both β and a finite dimensional feature of the baseline. Later we shall give an example to show how this leads to the test/confidence interval for a parameter that is defined through these two.

The baseline hazard is an arbitrary function and thus of infinite dimension. On the other hand, the hypothesis we will deal with is for finite dimensional parameters. Therefore, we introduce a new, finite dimensional parameter of the baseline hazard as

$$\theta = \int g(t)d\Lambda_0(t) \tag{4.10}$$

where $\Lambda_0(t)$ is the baseline cumulative hazard function and $g(t)$ is a given function. This may represent the cumulative hazard at a given time point, or the difference of the cumulative hazard at two time points, etc., depending on the choice of $g(t)$. The function $g(t)$ can even be multi-dimensional: $g(t) = (g_1(t),\ldots g_k(t))$. We shall call the new parameter θ the (finite dimensional) feature of the baseline hazard.

Since the confidence region can be obtained by inverting a test, we begin by describing how to test β and θ jointly. The hypothesis we first deal with involves both β and θ:

$$H_0 : \beta = \beta^* \quad \text{and} \quad \theta = \theta^* . \tag{4.11}$$

The likelihood we use to construct the test is the empirical likelihood $LogLik_{emp}$ of (4.6). The reason we switch from the Cox partial likelihood to the empirical likelihood is obvious: the Cox partial likelihood does not explicitly involve the baseline and therefore cannot be used to make inferences about the baseline.

For testing the null hypothesis $\beta = \beta^*$ and $\theta = \theta^*$, the log empirical likelihood *ratio* can be computed as the difference of two log empirical likelihoods. The empirical likelihood in the denominator of the ratio is easier; it is the $LogLik_{emp}$ where we maximize over both the baseline hazard and β. As discussed in the previous section, this maximum is obtained when $\beta = \hat{\beta}_c$ and the baseline hazard is equal to the Breslow estimator, i.e., (4.7) with $\beta = \hat{\beta}_c$ there.

The empirical likelihood in the numerator is a little harder to obtain. By a Lagrange multiplier argument, using $\beta = \beta^*$ and $\theta = \theta^*$ as the two constraints, we can show that the constrained maximum is given by $LogLik_{emp}$ where β is fixed at the null value, i.e., $\beta = \beta^*$ and the baseline hazard takes the form $w_i = w_i(\beta^*, \lambda^*)$ defined below.

First, let

$$w_i(\beta^*, \lambda) = \frac{\delta_i}{\sum_j e^{\beta^* Z_j} I[t_j \geq t_i] + \lambda g(t_i)}, \tag{4.12}$$

where $\lambda g(t_i)$ is the inner product, if λ and g are multidimensional.

Second, define λ^* as the solution of the equation(s)

$$\sum_{i=1}^{n} g(t_i) w_i(\beta^*, \lambda) = \theta^*. \tag{4.13}$$

To recap the above two steps: we fix $\beta = \beta^*$ and solve (4.13) to get the value λ^*. From there we obtain the w_i values via (4.12) with $\lambda = \lambda^*$. Finally, we use (4.6) with $\beta = \beta^*$ and $w_i = w_i(\beta^*, \lambda^*)$. This gives the numerator of the empirical likelihood ratio.

Together with the denominator obtained earlier, we can now form the log empirical likelihood ratio, and we have the following Wilks theorem for the null distribution of the log empirical likelihood ratio.

Theorem 35 *Assume the standard regularity conditions for the Cox model. Also assume the function $g(t)$ used to define parameter θ is such that $\int g(t) d\hat{\Lambda}_0(t)$ has finite positive variance, where $\hat{\Lambda}_0$ is the Breslow estimator.*

Under the null hypothesis H_0 in (4.11), as $n \to \infty$,

$$-2\{\log Lik_{emp}(\beta^*, w_i = w_i(\beta^*, \lambda^*)) - \log Lik_{emp}(\hat{\beta}_c, w_i = w_i(\hat{\beta}_c, 0))\} \longrightarrow \chi^2_{(q)}$$

in distribution, where $q = dim(\beta) + dim(\theta)$.

PROOF: Use the joint normality of $\hat{\beta}_c$ and the Breslow baseline estimator. See Zhou [139] for similar calculations. □

The λ^* value in the above calculation of $\log Lik_{emp}$ has a one-to-one mapping to the θ^* values via (4.13). Intuitively, the value of λ controls the amount of tilting of the baseline hazard in the direction of $g(\cdot)$. The λ^* is just the right amount of tilting so that the feature θ equals the value required by null hypothesis θ^*. When $\lambda = 0$, there is no tilting at all.

We can also specify the hypothesis in terms of β and λ. In other words, the following two hypotheses are identical:

$$H_0 : \beta = \beta^*, \quad \theta = \theta^* \tag{4.14}$$

and

$$H_0 : \beta = \beta^*, \quad \lambda = \lambda^*. \tag{4.15}$$

The empirical likelihood ratio test for a hypothesis in terms of β, λ is easier to calculate (we do not need to solve (4.13)). We provide an R function CoxEL that calculates the empirical likelihood ratio test for this form of the hypothesis (given β^* and λ^*), with the corresponding θ^* value included in the output. If you prefer the hypothesis in terms of β^* and θ^*, you must solve (4.13) first and then calculate the empirical likelihood using β^* and λ^*.

For example, the hypothesis $H_0 : \beta = \beta^*$ and $\lambda = 0$ is identical to $H_0 : \beta = \beta^*$ and $\theta = \sum g(t_i) w_i(\beta^*, 0)$. Recall that $w_i(\beta^*, 0)$ is the NPMLE of the baseline (Breslow) given $\beta = \beta^*$. In other words, $\lambda = 0$ corresponds to the case where no constraint is put on θ; thus the above two hypotheses are identical to the simpler hypothesis $H_0 : \beta = \beta^*$. For other values of λ^*, see examples below.

The value of λ controls the degree of tilting (i.e., deviation from NPMLE) of the baseline; a zero λ indicates no tilt of the baseline, i.e., the baseline is just the NPMLE.

In the R function CoxEL(), provided in the package ELYP, we input the hypothesized values β^*, λ^* and g function. The log empirical likelihood, $\log Lik_{emp}(\beta^*, w_i = w_i(\beta^*, \lambda^*))$, is computed for us, along with the corresponding θ^* value. Thus the function is best suited for testing hypotheses about β and λ jointly, but we shall see below that the function can also be used to test other hypotheses about β and θ.

Example 18 *Using the* smallcell *data from the* emplik *package as an example, we first find the NPMLE of the Cox model. Since it is the same as the maximum partial likelihood estimator, this can be computed by the* coxph( ) *function from the* survival *package.*

```
library(survival)
library(emplik)
data(smallcell)
coxph(Surv(survival, indicator)~arm, data=smallcell)
```

From the output of the coxph( ) *function we see the maximum partial likelihood estimator (which is also the NPMLE) of β is $\hat{\beta}_c = 0.5337653$. We next compute the two empirical likelihood values and then the likelihood ratio.*

```
library(ELYP)
myy <- smallcell$survival
myd <- smallcell$indicator
myZ <- smallcell$arm
myfun <- function(t){as.numeric(t <= 300)}
ELHa <- CoxEL(y=myy, d=myd, Z=myZ, beta=0.5337653,
                       lam=0, fun=myfun)$logEmpLik
temp <- CoxEL(y=myy,d=myd,Z=myZ,beta=0.5,lam=8,fun=myfun)
ELH0 <- temp$logEmpLik
temp$mu
## [1] 0.1676888
-2*(ELH0 - ELHa)
## [1] 0.1017061
```

From the output we see that the test of hypothesis

$$H_0 : \beta = 0.5, \ \lambda = 8$$

gives a -2 log empirical likelihood ratio 0.1017061. This corresponds to a p-value much larger than 0.05, using a chi square distribution with 2 degrees of freedom.

The above hypothesis can also be written as

$$H_0 : \beta = 0.5, \ \Lambda_0(300) = 0.1676888.$$

This is calculated as follows. As we can see from the output temp *of the function* CoxEL, *the* mu *value corresponding to $\lambda = 8$ is 0.1676888. And the definition of θ is $\int_0^\infty I[s \leq 300] d\Lambda_0(s) = \Lambda_0(300)$. In other words, $\theta = mu$ here implies $\Lambda_0(300) = 0.167888$.*

The NPMLE of $\Lambda_0(300)$ can be obtained by putting $\lambda = 0$ and $\beta = Cox$ maximum partial likelihood estimator:

```
CoxEL(y=myy, d=myd, Z=myZ, beta=0.5337653,
                      lam=0, fun=myfun)$mu
```

and in this case the NPMLE is 0.1737539.

If we want to test a hypothesis about β alone, for example,

$$H_0 : \beta = 0 ,$$

we may proceed as follows.

```
ELHa <- CoxEL(y=myy, d=myd, Z=myZ, beta=0.5337653,
                      lam=0, fun=myfun)$logEmpLik
ELH0 <- CoxEL(y=myy, d=myd, Z=myZ, beta=0,
                      lam=0, fun=myfun)$logEmpLik
-2*(ELH0 - ELHa)
```

This gives a chi square statistic of 6.838715. This is exactly the same as the partial likelihood ratio test given by the coxph( ) *function. According to the remark after Theorem 33, this should be the case. Here, since both* lam*'s are set to zero, the function defined by* fun *does not affect the outcome. Also, no restrictions on the baseline were imposed.*

If, on the other hand, we want to test the hypothesis $H_0 : \beta = 0.5, \theta = \Lambda_0(300) = 0.2$, then we need to do the following.

```
tempfun <- function(t, y, d, Z, b, fun, theta) {
muT <- CoxEL(y=y, d=d, Z=Z, beta=b, lam=t, fun=fun)$mu
return(theta - muT)
}
uniroot(f=tempfun, interval=c(-20,0),
        y=myy, d=myd, Z=myZ, b=0.5, fun=myfun, theta=0.2)
## $root
```

```
## [1] -15.9442
##
## $f.root
## [1] -3.865539e-09
##
## $iter
## [1] 4
##
## $estim.prec
## [1] 6.103516e-05
```

Here the `interval` input for the `uniroot` function defines where to search for the root, and it requires some adjustment: (1) we know the NPMLE of $\Lambda_0(300) = 0.1737539$ from the above results and we are testing $\Lambda_0(300) = 0.2$, a larger value than the NPMLE. This implies the solution of λ is negative, because $\Lambda_0(300)$ is a decreasing function in λ. (2) It is safer to use a small interval initially due to feasibility issues. If no solution is found, then we try larger intervals. This strategy is to avoid venturing into the *nonfeasible region* of λ, as discussed in Chapter 2 and Chapter 6.

This calculation tells us that testing $H_0 : \beta = 0.5, \Lambda_0(300) = 0.2$ is equivalent to testing $H_0 : \beta = 0.5, \lambda = -15.9442$. Now we can carry out this test as before.

4.2.4 Confidence Intervals for $h(\beta, \theta)$ or $h(\beta, \lambda)$

For a given dataset, the joint confidence region for β and λ can be obtained by inverting the hypothesis test (4.15) using the `CoxEL( )` function, as illustrated in the above examples. But often the interest is not in the confidence region/interval involving λ, β; rather, the interest is in the confidence region/interval for a quantity involving both β and $\Lambda_0(\cdot)$, or β and θ. We recall $\theta = \int g(t)d\Lambda_0(t)$.

Due to the invariance property of the confidence regions produced by inverting the likelihood ratio tests, we can easily translate the confidence region for β, λ into a confidence interval for a new parameter defined via both β and θ. We also note that θ is a monotone function of λ for any fixed β.

Next we offer an example that shows how to translate the confidence region for both β and λ jointly into a confidence interval for a one-dimensional parameter $\eta = h(\beta, \theta)$, where $h(\cdot, \cdot)$ is any continuous function.

We start with a confidence region for two parameters jointly: (β, λ): $\{\beta, \lambda : -2\log ELR(\beta, \lambda) < C\}$. Let us call this region U.

Next we transform the region U into a region for β, θ: $\{(\beta, \theta) : (\beta, \lambda) \in U\}$. Let us call this region $U2$.

Finally, we compute the collection $Uh = h(\beta, \theta)$, with all $(\beta, \theta) \in U2$. The confidence interval for $h(\beta, \theta)$ is just $[\min(Uh), \max(Uh)]$.

Example 19 *Using the* `smallcell` *data, we fit a Cox model and find a 95% confidence interval for* $\eta = [e^\beta - 1]\Lambda_0(300)$.

```
library(survival)
library(ELYP)
data(smallcell)
names(smallcell)    ## to see what variable the data include
coxph(Surv(survival, indicator)~arm, data=smallcell)
## from here we see beta(MLE) is 0.5337653, with SD=0.203
myy <- smallcell$survival
myd <- smallcell$indicator
myZ <- smallcell$arm
myfun <- function(t){as.numeric(t <= 300)}
CoxEL(y=myy, d=myd, Z=myZ, beta=0.5337653, lam=0,
                             fun=myfun)$logEmpLik
## [1] -500.8937
## this gives the max that logEmpLik can achieve
```

Next we find all the parameters (β and λ combinations) where the corresponding logEmpLik *is larger than or equal to* -502.8137. *(This value is obtained by* $-500.8937 - \chi^2(0.95, df = 1)/2$.) *Notice here that we use degree of freedom one, not two, since the final confidence interval is one-dimensional.*

Now we define the β range and λ range, whose combination will be searched for the maximum/minimum of η, while keeping the logEmpLik *larger than or equal to* -502.8137.

We define a vector of β values called bvec *and a vector of λ values called* lvec, *both of length 100. They will be our search domain.*

```
bvec <- 1:100/110 + 0.06
lvec <- (1:100)*1.3 - 50

myEtafun <- function(beta,theta){(exp(beta) - 1)*theta}
LLout1 <- LLout2 <- LLout3 <- matrix(NA, 100,100)

for(i in 1:100)for(j in 1:100) {
  temp <- CoxEL(y=myy, d=myd, Z=myZ, beta=bvec[i],
                               lam=lvec[j],fun=myfun)
  LLout1[i,j] <- temp$logEmpLik
  LLout2[i,j] <- temp$mu
  LLout3[i,j] <- myEtafun(beta=bvec[i], theta=temp$mu)
}

contour(bvec, lvec, z=LLout1, level=(-500.8937 - 3.84/2),
        xlab="beta", ylab="lambda", main="logEL and Eta")
par(new=TRUE)
contour(bvec, lvec, z=LLout3)

myIndex <- (LLout1 >= (-500.8937 - 3.84/2))
```

logEL and Eta

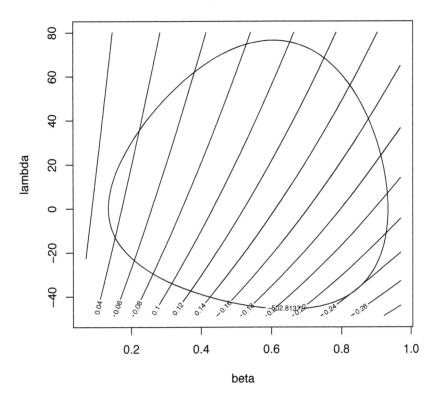

Figure 4.1: Confidence region of possible (β, λ) values and η contour lines over it.

```
max( LLout3[myIndex] )
## [1] 0.240251
min( LLout3[myIndex] )
## [1] 0.03054699
```

The range of the search, β vector bvec *and λ vector* lvec *above, is admittedly set by trial and error. The ideal range will cover the contour (a confidence region) shown in Fig. 4.1 below, but not much more (to save computational time). Also, if we search too far away from the contour, which is centered at $\beta = \hat{\beta}_c, \lambda = 0$, we may encounter the "feasibility" problem. Fig. 4.1 shows the joint confidence region for β and λ, and on top of that, the contour lines of $\eta = [e^\beta - 1]\Lambda_0(300)$.*

We can read from the plot the approximate values of the maximum and minimum of η over the confidence region of β and λ. By computing the max and min *of* LLout3 *over the confidence region we see that the 95% confidence interval for* $[e^\beta - 1]\Lambda_0(300)$ *is* $[0.03054699, 0.240251]$.

For Cox models with several βs, the search of the maximum and minimum of η over the confidence region becomes more challenging. We try to automate the search process, but currently the R function CoxFindL2( ) needs a nice input of StepSize to work.

```
CoxFindL2(BetaMLE=0.5337653, StepSize=c(0.05, 3),
          Efun=myEtafun, Hfun=myfun, y=myy, d=myd, Z=myZ)
## ......
## $Lower
## [1] 0.03061114
## ......
CoxFindU2(BetaMLE=0.5337653, StepSize=c(0.05, 3),
          Efun=myEtafun, Hfun=myfun, y=myy, d=myd, Z=myZ)
## ......
## $Upper
## [1] 0.2402764
## ......
```

The search method we used here is rather inefficient. But this method works for *any* function $h(\beta, \theta)$.

4.3   Confidence Band for the Baseline Cumulative Hazard

The Breslow estimator is the NPMLE of the baseline cumulative hazard function. It depends on $\hat{\beta}_c$, the maximum partial likelihood estimator of the regression parameter.

Confidence intervals for the baseline cumulative hazard at a fixed time point can be obtained as a special case of the $h(\beta, \theta)$ function, as in the previous example, by taking $\Lambda_0(a) = h(\beta, \theta) = \theta$, with the parameter θ defined as $\theta = \int I[s \le a]d\Lambda_0(s) = \Lambda_0(a)$.

Within a Cox model, the designation of the baseline hazard is somewhat arbitrary. For example, in the original model formulation, we designate the hazard of a (hypothetical) patient with all-zero covariates as the baseline; or we can designate the hazard of a patient with the average value of the covariate as the baseline (this approach is taken by SAS and R). Both conventions satisfy the Cox model, since the latter can be obtained by a shift transformation of the covariates. In the following discussion, we always assume the cumulative hazard function of interest is the one corresponding to covariates all equal to zero. As we see, this is always possible by a shift transformation of the covariates.

The simultaneous confidence intervals for the cumulative hazard function when time $t \in [a, b]$ is called a *confidence band*. Empirical likelihood can also be used to obtain such confidence bands for the baseline cumulative hazard function, which we briefly discuss below.

The problem of constructing a confidence band inside a Cox model is considered by Lin et al. [69]. Our presentation here is based on the use of the empirical likelihood ratio (see Zhu et al. [146]). The advantage of using empirical likelihood as opposed to a normal approximation used by Lin et al. [69] is that no transformation of the survival/hazard function is necessary before constructing the confidence band.

In the last section we discussed how to test

$$H_0 : \beta = \beta^*, \theta = \theta^*$$

or equivalently

$$H_0 : \beta = \beta^*, \lambda = \lambda^* .$$

Here we shall use a special definition $\theta^* = \int I[s \le t] d\Lambda_0(s) = \Lambda_0(t)$. For the time being, think of t as a fixed given time. We rewrite the hypothesis for this specific θ and emphasize its dependency on t by writing explicitly

$$H_0 : \beta = \beta^*, \theta(t) = \Lambda_0(t) .$$

Denote the empirical likelihood function, when we fix the two parameters at the above H_0, as

$$Lik_{emp}(\beta^*, w(\beta^*, \lambda^*)) .$$

The calculation of this EL is discussed just before Theorem 35.

The log empirical likelihood ratio for testing

$$H_0 : \theta(t) = \Lambda_0(t)$$

at a fixed t is then

$$W(t, \Lambda_0(t)) = -2\log \frac{\sup_{\beta, w}\{Lik_{emp}(\beta, w) \text{ subject to } \theta(t) = \Lambda_0(t)\}}{Lik_{emp}(\hat{\beta}_c, w(\hat{\beta}_c, \lambda = 0))} .$$

For fixed t, this log likelihood ratio has asymptotically a chi square distribution with one degree of freedom under H_0.

In order to construct a confidence band we shall, however, let t vary. Zhu et al. [146] includes the following theorem.

Theorem 36 *For $t \in [a,b]$ the test statistic $W(t, \Lambda_0(t))$ above, considered as a stochastic process, converges in distribution to $U^2(t)/v(t,t)$ in $D[a,b]$ as $n \to \infty$, where $U(t)$ is a mean-zero Gaussian process with variance-covariance function $v(s,t)$.*

The variance-covariance function $v(s,t)$ is defined by

$$v(s,t) = \sigma^2(\min(s,t)) + h(t)\Sigma^{-1}h^\top(s) ,$$

where Σ is the information matrix at β_0,

$$\sigma^2(t) = \int_0^t \frac{d\Lambda_0(s)}{z^{(0)}(\beta_0, s)} ,$$

and

$$h(t) = \int_0^t \frac{z^{(1)}(\beta_0,s)d\Lambda_0(s)}{z^{(0)}(\beta_0,s)} .$$

The functions $z^{(k)}(\beta_0,s)$ are defined in (4.20) and Section 4.7 at the end of this chapter includes an explicit definition of the information matrix.

One fact we see from the above theorem is that for any fixed t, $U^2(t)/v(t,t)$ is a random variable that has a chi square distribution with one degree of freedom. So this process generalizes the chi square random variable.

In order to set (for example) a 90% confidence level for the confidence band, we need to find C such that

$$P\left(\sup_{t\in[a,b]} \frac{|U(t)|}{\sqrt{v(t,t)}} < C\right) = 0.9 .$$

Once such C is found, the confidence band for the cumulative hazard over $[a,b]$ is then

$$\{(\Lambda_0(t),t) ; a \le t \le b \mid W(t,\Lambda_0(t)) < C^2\} .$$

There is no table for the tail probability of the process $U(t)/\sqrt{v(t,t)}$ over the interval $[a,b]$. But the distribution of this process can be simulated easily to set the confidence level of the band. For one such simulation set up, we refer readers to Lin et al. [69].

We give another simulation solution. Even though the Gaussian process $U(t)$ in the above theorem does not have independent increment, it can easily be simulated as follows.

Given a dataset, we notice that to construct the confidence band for $t \in [a,b]$, we only need to simulate the random vector $(U(t_i))$ where $t_i \in [a,b]$ and are observed survival values.

To this end, suppose $B(t)$ is a standard Brownian motion process. In addition, let G be a multivariate normal random vector with mean zero and variance covariance matrix Σ^{-1}, and independent of $B(t)$. It is not hard to show that for $\mathbf{t} = (t_i)$, where $t_i \in [a,b]$ and are observed survival values

$$\tilde{U}(\mathbf{t}) = h(\mathbf{t})^\top G + B(\sigma^2(\mathbf{t}))$$

have the same distribution as $U(\mathbf{t})$. Obviously $\tilde{U}(\mathbf{t})$ can be simulated easily.

See also Chapter 8, where other confidence bands are discussed. In particular, at the end of Section 8.3 we will discuss how to construct confidence bands for the ratio of two baseline cumulative hazards inside a stratified Cox model and comment further on the simulation of the limiting process.

Remark: In the above we discussed the construction of the confidence band for cumulative hazard by empirical likelihood. Due to the invariance property of empirical likelihood, this confidence band can easily be translated into a confidence band of a survival function. Indeed, a confidence band can be easily obtained for any quantity that is a monotone function of the cumulative hazard.

We plan to integrate the R code related to this computation into a future release of our package ELYP.

4.4 An Alternative Empirical Likelihood Approach

There is an alternative, simpler empirical likelihood approach to the Cox partial likelihood estimator. This approach starts with the estimating equation or score equation
(4.16) of the Cox partial likelihood estimator, $\ell(\beta) = \frac{\partial}{\partial \beta} \log Lik_{cox} = 0$. See Qin and
Jing [89].

In this context, we introduce the notation

$$\bar{z}_n^{(k)}(t, \beta_0) = \frac{1}{n} \sum_{j=1}^{n} I[T_j \geq t] z_j^{(k)} \exp(\beta_0 z_j) \quad \text{for } k = 0, 1, 2.$$

These are the weighted averages of the covariate moments.

A key result useful here is the martingale representation of the Cox score function
when the regression parameter β is fixed at the true value β_0:

$$\ell(\beta^0) = \sum_{i=1}^{n} \delta_i \left\{ z_i - \frac{\sum_{j=1}^{n} I[T_j \geq T_i] z_j \exp(\beta_0 z_j)}{\sum_{j=1}^{n} I[T_j \geq T_i] \exp(\beta_0 z_j)} \right\} \qquad (4.16)$$

$$= \sum_{i=1}^{n} \delta_i \left\{ z_i - \frac{\bar{z}_n^{(1)}(T_i, \beta_0)}{\bar{z}_n^{(0)}(T_i, \beta_0)} \right\} = \sum_{i=1}^{n} \int_0^{\infty} Q_{ni}(t) dI[T_i \leq t, \delta_i = 1], \qquad (4.17)$$

where

$$Q_{ni}(t) = z_i - \frac{\bar{z}_n^{(1)}(t, \beta_0)}{\bar{z}_n^{(0)}(t, \beta_0)}. \qquad (4.18)$$

After some (now standard) calculation, we can also verify that

$$\sum_{i=1}^{n} \int_0^{\infty} Q_{ni}(t) dI[T_i \leq t, \delta_i = 1] = \sum_{i=1}^{n} \int_0^{\infty} Q_{ni}(t) dM_i(t) \qquad (4.19)$$

where

$$M_i(t) = I[T_i \leq t, \delta_i = 1] - \int_0^t I[T_i \geq s] \lambda_i(s) ds$$

is the counting process martingale for the ith observation (with respect to a properly
defined filtration).

This is the well-known martingale representation of the score function from the
partial likelihood when $\beta = \beta_0$. For details, see the book by Kalbfleish and Prentice
[51], p. 173. We provide an outline in Section 2.10 of Chapter 2 to explain why the
$M_i(t)$ are martingales. One consequence of the martingale representation result is
that $E\ell(\beta_0) = 0$.

Now we focus on the martingale representation (4.19). We may argue that since
each term in the sum (4.19) is a martingale with respect to a properly defined filtration, therefore the empirical likelihood ratio Wilks theorem, i.e., Theorem 2 of
Chapter 1 applies (Martingale-difference version, uncensored data version).

Another way to arrive at the Wilks theorem is to notice that the functions $\bar{z}_n^1(t, \beta_0)$
and $\bar{z}_n^0(t, \beta_0)$ are averages of n terms. Under mild assumptions, for example, a random

design assumption (that z_i are i.i.d. random), they clearly converge to their expectations (e.g., by the law of large numbers) and the convergence is uniform in t by the Glivanko–Cantalli type theorem or by modern empirical process techniques.

Therefore, if we replace $\bar{z}_n^1(t, \beta_0)$ and $\bar{z}_n^0(t, \beta_0)$ by their limits, the error is negligible as $n \to \infty$. The following arguments are based on the fact that we can replace $\bar{z}_n^{(k)}(t, \beta_0)$, $k = 0, 1$ by their limits

$$z^{(k)}(t, \beta_0) = \lim_{n \to \infty} z_n^{(k)}(t, \beta_0). \tag{4.20}$$

The fact that these limits exist (law of large numbers) is the consequence of the regularity assumptions for the Cox model (see Assumption D at the end of this chapter) and the error

$$\sup_t |z^{(1)}(t, \beta_0) - \bar{z}_n^{(1)}(t, \beta_0)| = O_p(1/\sqrt{n}).$$

If we replace $\bar{z}_n^{(k)}(t, \beta_0)$ by its nonrandom limits, it is not hard to see that Equation (4.21) below is a sum of i.i.d. terms, at least under a random design assumption on the covariate z_i:

$$0 = \sum_{i=1}^n \int_0^\infty Q_i^*(t) dM_i(t) = \sum_{i=1}^n U(T_i, \delta_i, z_i) \quad \text{say}, \tag{4.21}$$

where $Q_i^*(t, \beta_0) = z_i - z^{(1)}(t, \beta_0)/z^{(0)}(t, \beta_0)$.

The empirical likelihood method with estimating equations involving a sum of i.i.d. terms has been treated by Owen [79] and Qin and Lawless [92]. Applying their empirical likelihood results to the estimating equations with i.i.d. terms, we immediately obtain an empirical likelihood ratio test for the Cox partial likelihood estimating equation.

We emphasize that here the estimating equation is in terms of the observation triplets (T_i, δ_i, z_i). The empirical likelihood corresponding to this sample of triplets (under random design) is just $\prod_{i=1}^n p_i$ (see Chapter 1), where p_i is the probability for the triplet. These triplets are completely observed and there is no censoring.

Remark: Here we assume the triplets $(T_i, \delta_i, z_i), i = 1, 2, \cdots, n$ are i.i.d. random vectors. These random vectors are *completely* observed and therefore the empirical likelihood for this random sample is just

$$EL = \prod_{i=1}^n p_i, \quad \text{and} \quad \sum_{i=1}^n p_i = 1 \tag{4.22}$$

and this EL is maximized when all $p_i = 1/n$. Here the probability p_i is the probability on the three-dimensional space for the random vector (T_i, δ_i, z_i). By contrast, in the first approach (Section 4.2) using empirical likelihood for the Cox model, the probability there is for the one-dimensional (potentially censored) lifetime random variable X_i.

Theorem 37 *Assume the covariates z_i in the Cox model are random and i.i.d. with a distribution that has finite variance. Assume also the regularity conditions for the Cox model A–D are satisfied. Then under the null hypothesis that*

$$H_0 : \beta = \beta_0 ,$$

we have, as $n \to \infty$,

$$-2\log\max_{p_i} \prod_{i=1}^{n} p_i n \xrightarrow{\mathcal{D}} \chi^2_{(p)}$$

where the maximization is taken over all p_i such that

$$p_i \geq 0; \quad \sum_{i=1}^{n} p_i = 1; \quad and \quad \sum_{i=1}^{n} p_i \left(\int Q_n(t) dM_i(t) \right) = 0 .$$

Remark: In the Cox model setting we have studied here, the two EL approaches in Sections 4.2 and 4.4 are asymptotically equivalent, in the sense that (1) they produce the same maximum empirical likelihood estimator and (2) the asymptotic power of the two resulting empirical likelihood ratio tests is the same. They are also equivalent to the Cox maximum partial likelihood estimator and the partial likelihood ratio test. But there is a crucial difference: the second approach hinges on the existence of an (efficient) estimating equation with asymptotically i.i.d. terms. In models other than the Cox model, deriving an efficient estimating equation with martingale terms is difficult.

The first EL approach seems more general, in that it does not assume the existence of an approximate i.i.d. estimating equation. Therefore, in the joint inference of β and baseline in the Cox model, and in the Yang and Prentice [129] extension of the Cox model we study next, we shall use the first EL approach.

4.5   Yang and Prentice Extension of the Cox Model

In the Cox model, the ratio of any two hazard functions is only a function of β and does not change over time t. But in reality, the ratio of treatment hazard and control hazard may change over time. For example, the benefit of a treatment may fade over time, or an initially harmful treatment may become beneficial over a longer time. Yang and Prentice [129] proposed an extension of the Cox model where the hazard ratio of treatment and control may change over time and the two hazards may even cross each other. They call this model the short-term/long-term hazard ratio model.

In the Yang and Prentice [129] model the hazard ratio of control to treatment is assumed to be

$$h_0(t)/h_i(t) = S_0(t)\exp(-\beta_1 z_i) + [1 - S_0(t)]\exp(-\beta_2 z_i) \qquad (4.23)$$

where $S_0(t) = \exp[-\Lambda_0(t)]$ is the baseline survival function, or the survival function for the patient with $z_i = 0$.

In the above model definition, if $t \to 0$, then $S_0(0) = 1$ and the ratio approaches $\exp(-\beta_1 z_i)$. When $t \to \infty$, the hazard ratio approaches $\exp(-\beta_2 z_i)$. Therefore,

$\exp(\beta_1 z_i)$ is called the short-term hazard ratio (of $h_i(t)$ to $h_0(t)$), and $\exp(\beta_2 z_i)$ the long-term.

In this model the hazard ratio is a convex combination of two constants: $\exp(-\beta_1 z_i)$ and $\exp(-\beta_2 z_i)$. The convex combination coefficient changes over time and is none other than the baseline survival probability at time t. This is to say that the hazard ratio changes monotonically from one constant (short-term) to a second constant (long-term). The speed of change is controlled by the change in the baseline survival probability.

Compared to the Cox model, this model has one more parameter: instead of one β, there are two βs. The draw back of this model is that the change of hazard ratio has to be monotone.

Clearly, the Yang and Prentice model includes the Cox proportional hazard model as a special case when the short-term and long-term β are equal. It also includes the proportional odds model as a special case when $\beta_2 = 0$. When the short-term and long-term β are of opposite sign, then the hazard functions of treatment and control cross each other.

The large sample property of the NPMLE in this model was studied by Diao et al. [20]. We shall discuss how to calculate the p-values and produce confidence regions/intervals using the empirical likelihood method here.

Using the Cox model EL treatment in Section 4.2 as a road map, we can and will try to go through the following points.

(1) Construct the empirical likelihood for the right censored observations, assuming they are generated from a Yang and Prentice (4.23) model. The empirical likelihood should involve both (short and long term) regression parameters and the baseline.

(2) In the empirical likelihood constructed in (1), hold β_1, β_2 fixed and maximize over the baseline hazard to obtain the "Breslow estimator" of the baseline.

(3) Plug the "Breslow estimator" back into the empirical likelihood to obtain the "partial likelihood," or, in this case, the profiled empirical likelihood to be more precise.

(4) Work with the EL constructed in (1). Treating β_1, β_2 and the baseline hazard simultaneously as parameters, test the hypothesis or find confidence regions for β_1, β_2 and a feature of the baseline hazard jointly.

(5) Finally, translate the confidence region obtained in (4) into a confidence interval for a one-dimensional parameter, defined by $h(\beta_1, \beta_2, \theta)$, where θ is a user-defined feature of the baseline hazard, $\theta = \int g(t) d\Lambda_0(t)$. We gave an example where the one-dimensional parameter of interest is the hazard ratio at a given time t_0.

The plan here is very similar to the treatment of the Cox model, except here the baseline estimator or "Breslow estimator" is not explicitly available, but needs to be computed iteratively. Hence the "partial likelihood" or profile EL is also not explicit.

Let us elaborate on step (1) above (constructing the empirical likelihood). Following along the lines of Section 4.2, starting with the contribution to empirical likelihood of a single right censored observation, but using the Yang and Prentice model instead of the Cox model, we see after simple calculation that the log empirical likelihood based on n independent observations (T_i, δ_i, Z_i), coming from a Yang and Prentice model, is

$$\log Lik(\beta_1, \beta_2, w_i) = \sum_{i=1}^{n} \delta_i \log \frac{e^{\beta_2 Z_i} w_i}{1 + (e^{(\beta_2 - \beta_1) Z_i} - 1) S_0(T_i)}$$

$$- e^{\beta_2 Z_i} \log[1 + e^{(\beta_1 - \beta_2) Z_i} \frac{1 - S_0(T_i)}{S_0(T_i)}] \qquad (4.24)$$

where we denoted $w_i = \Delta \Lambda_0(t_i)$. Also, recall $\Lambda_0(t) = \sum_{T_i \le t} w_i$, and $S_0(t) = \exp[-\Lambda_0(t)]$.

We notice that this log empirical likelihood reduces to the Cox model log empirical likelihood when $\beta_1 = \beta_2$ (not the partial likelihood but the empirical likelihood). (Exercise)

Now let us elaborate on step (2) above as well. The baseline estimator (the "Breslow estimator") can be obtained by taking a partial derivative of the log EL above with respect to w_i and setting it to zero. After some tedious but routine calculations, we have

$$w_k(\beta_1, \beta_2) = \frac{\delta_k}{- \sum_{i=1}^{n} g_i I[T_k \le T_i]} \qquad (4.25)$$

where g_i involves the baseline survival S_0 and regression parameters:

$$g_i = g_i(S_0(T_i)) = \frac{\delta_i S_0(T_i)[\exp(-\beta_1 Z_i) - \exp(-\beta_2 Z_i)] - 1}{\exp(-\beta_2 Z_i) + [\exp(-\beta_1 Z_i) - \exp(-\beta_2 Z_i)] S_0(T_i)} . \qquad (4.26)$$

Even when the two βs are known, Equations (4.25) and (4.26) do not give an explicit solution since both sides of Equation (4.25) depend on the unknown baseline. This naturally leads to an iterative algorithm: we start with a discrete baseline hazard/survival that has its jumps at the observed event times, and use it to compute (4.26). Then we plug the obtained g_i into the right-hand side of (4.25) and get an updated baseline hazard/survival at the left-hand side of (4.25).

Examples we have computed show that this iteration converges very quickly. We show a typical convergence below in a plot (Figure 4.2).

Example 20 *We take the dataset* ggas *from the R package ELYP and assume the survival times follow a Yang and Prentice model. For fixed β_1 and β_2, we plot the baseline hazard function using the iterative algorithm inspired by (4.25) and (4.26).*

```
library(ELYP)
data(GastricCancer)
ggas <- GastricCancer
temp <- fitYP41(Y=ggas[1,], d=ggas[2,], Z=ggas[4,],
                        beta1=1.81, beta2=-1)
plot( sort(ggas[1,]), exp(-cumsum(temp$BaselineH)) )
```

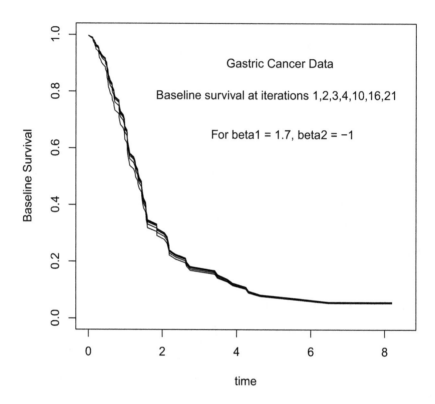

Figure 4.2: Calculation of the baseline survival function in the Yang and Prentice [129] model.

This will show the baseline survival estimator, when β_1 and β_2 are fixed at 1.81 and -1, respectively. We fix the βs at these values, because (as we shall see later) they are close to the NPMLEs of the two βs.

To show the convergence of the baseline estimator from (4.25) and (4.26) iteration, we deliberately set the number of iterations at low and fixed numbers. Result for the Gastric Cancer data is shown in Fig. 4.2. We also set the two βs at several different values and the resulting plots are similar. Simulated dataset with sample size ranging from 40 to 500 are also used. The convergence of the baseline are all similar to Fig. 4.2. An iteration number of 30 seems appropriate. We set a larger number (= 60) in fitYP41 as the default iteration number just to be sure for convergence.

The remaining steps (3), (4) and (5) are computation intensive. Readers might want consult Chapter 6 before reading the computation of these steps below.

Next, we find the NPMLE of β_1 and β_2. This is equivalent to finding the maximizer of the empirical likelihood (4.24), which is in the output of fitYP41( ) for the two βs, as in the previous example. We use the R function optim( ) to search for the maximizer. Other optimization function may also work.

```
myffitYP41 <- function(x, myY, myd, myZ) {
          x1 <- x[1]
          x2 <- x[2]
          tempT <- fitYP41(Y=myY, d=myd, Z=myZ, beta1=x1,
                                              beta2=x2)
          return( - tempT$EmpLik)
}


> optim(par = c(0, 0), fn=myffitYP41, myY=ggas[1,],
                       myd=ggas[2,], myZ=ggas[4,])
## $par
## [1]  1.816674 -1.002082
##
## $value
## [1] 383.3159
##
## $counts
## function gradient
##       61        NA
##
## $convergence
## [1] 0
##
## $message
## NULL
```

So, the NPMLE is $\hat{\beta}_1 = 1.816674$, $\hat{\beta}_2 = -1.002082$. Since the two βs are of opposite sign, the hazard ratio for the treatment and the control cross according to the Yang and Prentice model.

Step 4 is to test the hypothesis for the three parameters β_1, β_2, and θ, where θ is defined as

$$\theta = \int g(t)d\Lambda_0(t) ,$$

$\Lambda_0(t)$ is the baseline cumulative hazard and $g(t)$ is a user defined function.

Once we fix the $g(t)$ function, there is a one-to-one (monotone) correspondence between the parameter θ and a new parameter λ. This is similar to the case we discussed in Section 4.2.3, and $\lambda = 0$ always corresponds to $\theta = NPMLE$.

Therefore, we would rather test the hypothesis involving β_1, β_2 and λ, since this is easier than (but equivalent to) testing the hypothesis involving β_1, β_2 and θ. The R function fitYP3( ) can accomplish this. It is actually designed for models that have an extra parameter α. Here we do not have the parameter α in the model, so we just enter 0 for the first column of Z and 0 for the first parameter value of the vector βs in the following R code.

Also note that in this example we take $g(t)$ to be the indicator function: $g(t) = I[t \leq 1.5]$.

The following calculations test

$$H_0 : \beta_1 = 1.8, \ \beta_2 = -1, \ \lambda = 1 \ .$$

```
fitYP3(Y=ggas[1,], d=ggas[2,], Z=cbind(0, ggas[4,]),
            beta1=c(0, 1.8), beta2=c(0, -1), lam=1,
            fun=function(x){as.numeric(x <=1.5)} )
## $LogEmpLik
## [1] -383.3276
##
## $MuLam
## [1] 0.8281782
##
## $BaseHazw
##    [1] 0.003117123 0.003126870 0.003330146 ...
## ...
```

This gives a log empirical likelihood value of -383.3276 when the three parameters are fixed at the hypothesized values. In order to determine the p-value for H_0, we must also find the maximum of the log empirical likelihood when there is no restriction on the three parameters. This corresponds to $\beta_1 = 1.816674$, $\beta_2 = -1.002082$ and $\lambda = 0$, since these are the NPMLEs.

```
fitYP3(Y=ggas[1,], d=ggas[2,], Z=cbind(0,ggas[4,]),
        beta1=c(0, 1.816674), beta2=c(0, -1.002082),
        lam=0, fun=function(x){as.numeric(x <=1.5)})
## $LogEmpLik
## [1] -383.3159
##
## $MuLam
## [1] 0.8495497
## ...
```

We can now calculate the -2 log empirical likelihood ratio: $-2 \times (-383.3276 - -383.3159) = 0.0234$, which is not significant on the chi square distribution with 3 degrees of freedom (p-value = 0.999).

Another thing we can infer from the output is that the θ value corresponding to $\lambda = 0$ (when $\beta_1 = 1.816674, \beta_2 = -1.002082$) is 0.8495497 (MuLam in the output).

The 90% joint confidence region for β_1, β_2 and λ can be described as all those triplets such that fitYP3( ) will return a LogEmplik value larger than $\chi^2_{(3)}(0.9)/2 - 383.3159$, because those values will lead to -2 log empirical likelihood ratios less than qchisq(0.90, df=3) = 6.251389.

The above calculation of the p-value (from -2 log empirical likelihood ratio =

0.0234) merely indicates that the triplet $\beta_1 = 1.8$, $\beta_2 = -1$, $\lambda = 1$ is inside the confidence region. Or equivalently, the triplet $\beta_1 = 1.8, \beta_2 = -1, \theta = 0.8281782$ is inside the 90% joint confidence region. How to picture the three-dimensional confidence region as a whole is difficult.

Finally, we show how to find confidence intervals for a one-dimensional parameter defined by a function $h(\beta_1, \beta_2, \lambda)$ or $h(\beta_1, \beta_2, \theta)$.

To illustrate the idea, we find the confidence interval for the (treatment/control) hazard ratio at time $t = 1.5$. By the Yang and Prentice model this ratio at $t = 1.5$ is (control: $Z = 0$, treatment: $Z = 1$):

$$h_0(1.5)/h_1(1.5) = S_0(1.5)\exp(-\beta_1) + [1 - S_0(1.5)]\exp(-\beta_2)$$

where S_0 is the baseline survival function. Recall $S_0(t) = \exp[-\Lambda_0(t)]$. The ratio of treatment to control is then

$$h_1(1.5)/h_0(1.5) = \frac{1}{S_0(1.5)\exp(-\beta_1) + [1 - S_0(1.5)]\exp(-\beta_2)} \,. \qquad (4.27)$$

We need to search inside the three-dimensional confidence region of β_1, β_2, and λ to find the largest and smallest value of the ratio (4.27), which is a function of $(\beta_1, \beta_2, S_0(1.5))$ and thus is also a function of $(\beta_1, \beta_2, \Lambda_0(1.5))$ which in turn is a function of $(\beta_1, \beta_2, \lambda)$ because $\Lambda_0(1.5)$ and λ have a 1 to 1 correspondence, after we picked $g(t) = I[t \le 1.5]$. We define the function $g(t) = I[t \le 1.5]$ inside myLLfun( ).

The code below is for finding the confidence interval for the parameter $h_1(1.5)/h_0(1.5)$ inside the Yang and Prentice model. The Pfun( ) and myLLfun( ) are already defined inside the package ELYP. The function Pfun( ) computes the ratio (4.27). The function myLLfun( ) computes the empirical likelihood, given three parameters. However, the supplied myLLfun( ) uses a $g(t)$ function $I[t \le 0.25]$. We want $g(t) = I[t \le 1.5]$, hence we define a function myLLfun1.5 below.

We need to find the maximum and minimum values of the parameter (4.27) over the three-dimensional region U for β_1, β_2 and λ, where U is the region such that the log empirical likelihood (as a function of these three parameters) is larger than $MAX - 3.84/2$. Again, the chi square threshold 3.84 is from the chi square with *one* degree of freedom and the desired 95% coverage probability for the confidence interval, since we eventually are getting a one-dimensional confidence interval.

```
myLLfun1.5 <- function(mle, dataMat) {
                    myLLfun(mle, dataMat,
                    fun=function(x){as.numeric(x <= 1.5)})
                    }
findU3(NPmle=c(1.816674, -1.002082), ConfInt=c(1.2,0.5,10),
            LogLikfn=myLLfun1.5, Pfun=Pfun, dataMat=ggas)

## ...
## $Upper
## [1] 1.091503
```

```
## ...

findL3(NPmle=c(1.816674, -1.002082), ConfInt=c(1.2,0.5,10),
          LogLikfn=myLLfun1.5, Pfun=Pfun, dataMat=ggas)
## ...
## $Lower
## [1] 0.3445221
## ...
```

From the output, we see that the 95% confidence interval for $h_1(1.5)/h_0(1.5)$ is $[0.3445221, 1.091503]$.

The ConfInt input of the findU3( ) should be approximately a half length of the 95% confidence interval for β_1, β_2 and λ, respectively. These only need to be approximate values, used to determine the initial search area. Otherwise the search may need more steps and become slower. The default confidence level is 95%. If we would rather compute the 90% confidence interval, we need to add level=qchisq(0.9, df=1) to the functions findU3( ) and findL3( ).

4.6 Historical Notes

The equivalency of the profiled empirical likelihood and the partial likelihood (Theorem 33) was noted by Johansen [50].

The joint asymptotic normality of the Cox estimator $\hat{\beta}_c$ and the Breslow estimator was studied by Tsiatis [116], among others.

Nonproportional hazards in the Cox model is a hot topic. The most common way to handle nonproportional hazards is to include a time change covariate $z(t)$ in the Cox model. The drawback is that the form of the change in hazards ratio are all pre-specified in the covariate. For example, the time point where the hazards ratio change from above one to below one must be specified in $z(t)$. On the other hand, the short-term/long-term hazard ratio model of Yang and Prentice do not need to specify a time change $z(t)$. The time change hazards ratio in the Yang–Prentice model is determined by the baseline survival function, which in turn is an infinitely dimensional (nonparametric) parameter.

Zhou [139] investigated the case where there is some finite dimensional information about the baseline available for the Cox model. He showed the baseline information can improve the estimation of β.

4.7 Some Known Results about the Cox Model

We list here without proof some useful results about the Cox model partial likelihood and maximum partial likelihood estimator, especially its large sample property. Theorem 34 in Section 4.2 made use of this result to derive the asymptotic chi square distribution for the -2 log empirical likelihood ratio.

Detailed proof can be found in Kalbfleisch and Prentice [51] or Fleming and Harrington [28] using counting process martingale theories.

Using the definition of log partial likelihood $\log Lik_{cox}$ given in (4.5), we define the score function and the information matrix based on the log partial likelihood as

$$\ell(\beta) = \frac{\partial}{\partial \beta} \log Lik_{cox}$$

and

$$I(\beta) = \frac{\partial^2}{(\partial \beta)^2} \log Lik_{cox}.$$

Definition: If $\hat{\beta}_c$ is the solution of the above score equation, i.e., $\ell(\hat{\beta}_c) = 0$, then $\hat{\beta}_c$ is called the Cox partial likelihood estimator of the regression coefficient.

Theorem 38 *(Andersen and Gill [4]) Under mild regularity conditions A–D below, we have the following results:*

(1) If $\beta_n^\star$ is a sequence of consistent estimators, i.e., $\beta_n^\star \xrightarrow{P} \beta_0$, then

$$\frac{1}{n} I(\beta_n^\star) \xrightarrow{P} \Sigma.$$

(2) If $\hat{\beta}_c$ is the solution of the score equation above, $\ell(\hat{\beta}_c) = 0$, then, as $n \to \infty$,

$$\sqrt{n}(\hat{\beta}_c - \beta_0) \xrightarrow{D} N(0, \Sigma^{-1}), \tag{4.28}$$

where the invertibility of Σ is part of assumption D.

A. (Finite hazard on finite interval) $\int_0^\tau \lambda_0(t)dt < \infty$ for $\tau < \infty$.

B. (Asymptotic stability of design) There exists a neighborhood $\mathcal{B}$ of β_0 and scalar, vector and matrix functions $z^{(0)}(\beta,t)$, $z^{(1)}(\beta,t)$, and $z^{(2)}(\beta,t)$ defined on $\mathcal{B} \times [0,\tau]$ such that for $k = 0,1,2$

$$\sup_{t \in [0,\tau], \beta \in \mathcal{B}} \|z_n^{(k)}(\beta,t) - z^{(k)}(\beta,t)\| \xrightarrow{P} 0.$$

We comment that these conditions are automatically satisfied if we assume the covariates z_i are i.i.d. and bounded.

C. There exists $\delta > 0$ such that

$$n^{-1/2} \sup_{i,t} |Z_i(t)| Y_i(t) I_{[\beta_0' Z_i(t) > -\delta |Z_i(t)|]} \xrightarrow{P} 0.$$

D. (Asymptotic regularity conditions) Let $\mathcal{B}$, $z^{(k)}$, $k = 0,1,2$, be as in Condition B and define $e = s^{(1)}/s^{(0)}$ and $v = s^{(2)}/s^{(0)} - e^{\otimes 2}$. For all $\beta \in \mathcal{B}, t \in [0,1]$:

$$s^{(1)}(\beta,t) = \frac{\partial}{\partial \beta} s^{(0)}(\beta,t), \quad s^{(2)}(\beta,t) = \frac{\partial^2}{\partial \beta^2} s^{(0)}(\beta,t),$$

$s^{(0)}(\cdot,t)$, $s^{(1)}(\cdot,t)$, and $s^{(2)}(\cdot,t)$ are continuous functions of $\beta \in \mathcal{B}$, uniformly in $t \in$

$[0,1]$, $s^{(0)}$, $s^{(1)}$, and $s^{(2)}$ are bounded on $\mathcal{B} \times [0,1]$; $s^{(0)}$ is bounded away from zero on $\mathcal{B} \times [0,1]$, and the matrix

$$\Sigma = \int_0^\tau v(\beta_0,t)s^{(0)}(\beta_0,t)\lambda_0 dt$$

is positive definite.

The notation in Conditions A–D is well defined in Andersen and Gill [4].

4.8 Exercises

Exercise 4.1 *Suppose $Y_1, Y_2, \cdots, Y_n$ are independent exponential random variables with the parameter $\lambda_i = \exp(\beta Z_i)$. Suppose also that $g(t)$ is an arbitrary, monotone increasing function with $g(0) = 0$. Show that $g(Y_1), \cdots, g(Y_n)$ follow a Cox proportional hazards model. What is the baseline hazard function here?*

Exercise 4.2 *Verify that the Yang and Prentice model (4.23) reduces to the proportional odds model when $\beta_2 = 0$.*

Exercise 4.3 *Verify that the log empirical likelihood (4.24) reduces to the Cox model log empirical likelihood when $\beta_1 = \beta_2$ (not the partial likelihood but the empirical likelihood).*

Exercise 4.4 *Assume $M_i(t)$ are martingales. Verify the following fact: if we replace the upper limit, ∞, of the integral in (4.19) by τ, then it is a martingale in τ. Hint: see Section 2.10 of Chapter 2.*

Exercise 4.5 *The stratified Cox model is an extension of the simple Cox model. The model assumes the sample can be divided into k mutually exclusive groups and each group has its own arbitrary baseline hazard function. However, all groups share the same multiplicative treatment effect (β).*

The model assumes that the hazard function for survival times $Y_{ij}; i = 1,2,\cdots,k; j = 1,2,\cdots,n_i$ of group i, with covariate z_{ij}, is given by

$$h_{ij}(t) = h_{i0}(t)\exp(\beta z_{ij}),$$

where $h_{i0}(t)$ is an arbitrary baseline hazard function for group i.

Derive the empirical likelihood for censored observations coming from this model. Verify a relation similar to Theorem 33 still holds.

Chapter 5

Empirical Likelihood Analysis of Accelerated Failure Time Models

Accelerated Failure Time (AFT) models are similar to classic linear regression models, except the responses are the log of the survival times, and more important, the responses are subject to censoring. We consider only right censoring here.

In statistical analysis outside of survival analysis, the classic linear model is one of the most widely used models and the least squares method is the most popular estimation method for such a model. The AFT model is a direct generalization of these to censored survival data analysis. It is widely viewed as an alternative regression model to the Cox model discussed in Chapter 4.

5.1 AFT Models

The semi-parametric accelerated failure time (AFT) model is an extension of the linear regression model to the analysis of survival data. The model assumption is that for survival times T_i, $i = 1, \cdots, n$,

$$\log(T_i) = Y_i = X_i^\top \beta + \varepsilon_i , \tag{5.1}$$

where the distribution $F_\varepsilon(\cdot)$ of the error term ε_i is unspecified (except for some location identification requirement such as mean zero or median zero). The X_i are the observed covariates, either fixed or random.

More important, the responses, Y_i or T_i, are subject to right censoring: that is, we observe only $Z_i = \min(Y_i, C_i)$ and $\delta_i = I[Y_i \leq C_i]$ for some censoring time variables C_i instead of Y_i. The distribution of C_i is also unspecified.

When the errors are i.i.d. and their distribution F_ε is assumed known, for example, the extreme value distribution, then the above model (5.1) becomes the parametric AFT model. Such models are quite well studied in survival analysis. The parametric likelihood of the censored data from this parametric AFT model is well-known (see, e.g., Klein and Moeschenberger [59]) and can be used for statistical inference. Most software packages include likelihood-based inference for the extreme value parametric AFT model and a few alternative error distributions. See SAS proc lifereg and R function survreg in the survival package. Note that the extreme value parametric AFT model is also called the Weibull regression model, due to the fact that the logarithm of a Weibull random variable is an extreme value random variable. The semi-parametric AFT models we study here, however, do not assume *any* particular error distribution. Therefore, the semi-parametric AFT model serves as a generalization of the extreme value parametric AFT model, by relaxing the assumption on the error distribution.

In the previous chapter dealing with the Cox model, we constructed the empirical likelihood on the responses Y_i or based on the estimating equations. Here, for AFT models, we have difficulty constructing empirical likelihood for the responses Y_i. The reason is clear if we suppose the distribution of responses are discrete. In a Cox model, the responses Y_i for different covariates have the same, fixed support. But in the AFT model, even with i.i.d. errors, the responses Y_i for different covariates *do not* have the same support (their support is a shift of each other).

Due to this difficulty, the empirical likelihood analysis for the semi-parametric AFT model has to be based on estimating equations. We saw one such estimating equation in Chapter 2 based on the (Gehan or log rank) rank test. Here we shall study estimators based on the (generalized) least squares estimating equations.

Remark: Weibull regression and the extreme value AFT model are actually the same model, except one is formulated with the original survival times and the other is formulated with the log transformation of the survival times. This fact is obvious to anyone who has used SAS proc lifereg: when you ask to fit an exponential/Weibull regression model, SAS returns an extreme value AFT model.

The Cox model generalizes the exponential regression model by dropping the exponential distribution assumption. Similarly, the semi-parametric AFT model generalizes the extreme value AFT model by dropping the extreme value distribution assumption. They are two different generalizations: one starts from the exponential regression formulation, the other starts from the log formulation of the exponential regression model.

Least squares estimating equations in the AFT model can take several different forms. The difference is mainly in how censoring is accommodated. We discuss two. Each is appropriate under its own set of assumptions. We first discuss in detail the model assumptions in the above AFT models. We distinguish two different types of data generating schemes under random right censoring: the accelerated failure time *regression* model and the accelerated failure time *correlation* model.

This differentiation is similar to that made by Freedman [29], in the bootstrap context, regarding linear models. In that case the difference also led to two different bootstrap strategies: re-sampling the residuals or re-sampling the cases. Owen [81] also discussed these two types of model assumption in the EL analysis.

Owen [80] recognized this difference with empirical likelihood for linear models. He suggested that the empirical likelihood should be constructed based on the homoscedasticity of the (Y_i, X_i) vector for *correlation* models, while the empirical likelihood should be constructed based on the homoscedasticity of the errors e_i for *regression* models. Although they have different interpretations, the two empirical likelihoods in Owen [80] look the same:

$$\prod_{i=1}^{n} p_i \quad \text{where} \quad \sum_{i=1}^{n} p_i = 1 \,.$$

We find that the difference in AFT models is more profound, due to censoring. First, in the AFT model, different data-generation models require different estimating equations (i.e., least squares equations but with different ways to account for censoring). Second, different AFT models call for different definitions of the censored empirical likelihood function. Third, different assumptions on the censoring times C_i are required for the two types of AFT model.

Next, we discuss the distinction between the empirical likelihood functions for AFT models under random right censoring. We call those EL based on the i.i.d. of vectors (Y_i, X_i) the *case-wise* EL, and those EL based on the i.i.d. of error terms the *residual-wise* EL.

It is perhaps beneficial to note how the bootstrap treats these two different regression models: we re-sample the (Y_i, X_i) cases for the correlation models, and we re-sample the residuals for the regression models.

Without censoring, the two different likelihood formulations yield similar likelihood functions and produce identical p-values and confidence regions, although interpreted differently and valid under different assumptions (see Owen [80]). With censoring, however, the *case-wise* empirical likelihood is quite different from the *residual-wise* empirical likelihood, and their respective estimates, p-values and confidence regions are different.

5.2 AFT Regression Models

The regression model is appropriate when the measurement error of the response is the main source of uncertainty (Freedman [29]). The true value of the p-dimensional parameter vector β solves $\int (y - x^\top \beta) x \, dF_e = 0$, where F_e denotes the error distribution. The main assumptions in the regression model are

(i) the covariates, $x_1, \cdots, x_n$, are row vectors of p-dimensional fixed constants, forming a matrix of full rank;

(ii) the errors, $e_1, \cdots, e_n$, are independent, with common distribution F_e having mean 0 and finite variance σ^2 (both F_e and σ^2 unknown);

(iii) the censoring time variables, $C_1, \cdots, C_n$, are independent with a common, unknown distribution G and independent of Y_i conditionally on x_i.

Popular estimators of the parameter vector β in this model with censored data include the Buckley–James estimator (Buckley and James [10], Lai and Ying [64]) and rank-based estimators (see Chapter 7 of Kalbfleisch and Prentice [51]) and references therein; also see Jin et al. [47]).

The following empirical likelihood approach to the Buckley–James estimator was proposed by Zhou and Li [142]. They proposed that the empirical likelihood be constructed based on the residuals, and also that the Buckley–James estimating function be rewritten in terms of residuals. Let

$$Z_i = \min(Y_i, C_i) \quad \text{and} \quad \delta_i = I_{[Y_i \le C_i]} \,.$$

Let b be a (length p) vector, and define the *residuals* with respect to b as

$$e_i(b) = Z_i - x_i^\top b .$$

5.3 The Buckley–James Estimator

Before we construct the empirical likelihood, let us digress to discuss the Buckley–James estimator and its related estimating equations.

The Buckley–James estimator of β is the solution to the estimating equations

$$0 = \sum_{i=1}^n \left\{ \delta_i e_i(b) + (1 - \delta_i) \sum_{j:e_j>e_i} \frac{e_j(b)\Delta\hat{F}(e_j)}{1 - \hat{F}(e_i)} \right\} X_i , \qquad (5.2)$$

where $\hat{F}(\cdot)$ is the Kaplan–Meier estimator computed from the residuals $(e_i(b), \delta_i)$. We notice the summation term inside the curly bracket is an estimation of the conditional expectation, $\hat{E}(Y_i - X_i b | Z_i, \beta = b, \delta_i = 0)$, using a discrete distribution.

The above equation is similar to the ordinary least squares estimating equation for β (when there is no censoring),

$$0 = \sum_{i=1}^n (Y_i - x_i^\top b) X_i = \sum_{i=1}^n e_i(b) X_i .$$

The idea behind the Buckley–James estimating equation (5.2) is to replace the residuals, when they are censored, by their (estimated) conditional expectations. The estimation of the conditional expectation is done in terms of the residual time scale, since the error terms are assumed i.i.d. And the error distribution is estimated non-parametrically by the Kaplan–Meier estimator.

The estimating equation (5.2) is, unfortunately, implicit in b and therefore requires an iterative algorithm to solve for the Buckley–James estimator. Another problem with the estimating equation is that it is not constructed according to e_i but to y_i or the conditional expectation of y_i. Consequently, the ith term of (5.2) involves not only e_i but also all the e_j's, where $e_j > e_i$. Recall our assumption is that the error terms are i.i.d. This makes the terms in (5.2) correlated and makes the empirical likelihood hard to construct.

We shall rewrite the estimating equation in a form that is easier to analyze. There are two summation signs in the Buckley–James estimating equation (5.2); one is for index i and the other is for index j. Exchanging the order of the summations, we have

$$0 = \sum_{j=1}^n \delta_j e_j(b) \left\{ X_j + \sum_{i:e_i<e_j,\delta_i=0} \frac{X_i \Delta\hat{F}(e_j)}{1 - \hat{F}(e_i)} \right\} . \qquad (5.3)$$

The jth term in this form of Buckley–James estimating equation involves e_j and e_i's where $e_i < e_j$.

For people familiar with the counting process martingale theory, whether the e_i's are before or after the current time $t = e_j$ (i.e., history or future) makes a critical difference: we may say that the e_i's for $e_i < e_j$ are *predictable*, since they are contained in the growing history information filtration $\mathcal{F}$ of ordered e_j's. In other words, imagining that the time t is going from the smallest e_j to the largest e_j, the terms in (5.3) involve the current e_j and the history at time e_j, but not the future.

The terms in this second form of the Buckley–James estimating equation are similar to martingales. This second form will be used in several places later.

Zhou and Li [142] proposed that empirical likelihood be formulated with respect to the (right censored) residuals $(e_i(b), \delta_i)$ as follows: given b, the *residual-wise* empirical likelihood for some univariate distribution F (of error) is defined as

$$EL_e(F) = \prod_{\delta_i=1} p_i \prod_{\delta_i=0} \left(1 - \sum_{e_j(b) \leq e_i(b)} p_j\right), \qquad (5.4)$$

where $p_i = dF[e_i(b)]$ is the probability mass placed by F on the ith residual. The likelihood ratio is

$$R_e(b) = \frac{\sup\{EL_e(F)|F \in \mathbb{F}^b\}}{\sup\{EL_e(F)|F \in \mathfrak{F}\}}, \qquad (5.5)$$

where $\mathfrak{F}$ denotes the set of all univariate distributions that place positive probabilities on each uncensored $e_i(B)$, as $EL_e(F) = 0$ for any F that places zero probability on any uncensored $e_i(B)$; $\mathbb{F}^b$ denotes a subset of $\mathfrak{F}$ where $B = b$ and that satisfies the constraints

$$\sum_{i=1}^n p_i \delta_i e_i(b)\tilde{x}_i = 0 \qquad (5.6)$$

for

$$\tilde{x}_i = \frac{1}{\Delta\hat{F}(e_i)}\left\{X_i + \sum_{\delta_j=0, j:e_j<e_i} \frac{X_j \Delta\hat{F}(e_i)}{1 - \hat{F}(e_j)}\right\}.$$

We point out that, aside from the $\Delta\hat{F}(e_i)$ in the denominator, $\tilde{x}$ is just the expression inside the curly bracket in Equation (5.3), and thus Equation (5.6) is derived from (5.3). The reason to divide the probability $\Delta\hat{F}(e_i)$ is that the total weight inside the curly bracket is precisely proportional to $\Delta\hat{F}(e_i)$.

It is not hard to see that the EL in the denominator of (5.5) is maximized by $B = \hat{\beta}$, the Buckley–James estimator, and the Kaplan Meier estimator of the residuals $e_i(\hat{\beta})$, whose calculation is straightforward. Maximization calculation is required only for the numerator of (5.5). When $b = \hat{\beta}$, it is easy to see that the likelihood ratio $R_e(\hat{b}) = 1$ and thus the confidence regions based on (5.5) are "centered" at the Buckley–James estimator.

Zhou and Li [142] proved the following theorem.

Theorem 39 *Consider the AFT regression model (5.1) and the model assumptions we discussed in Section 5.2. When $b = \beta_0$, the residuals $e_i(\beta_0) = Y_i - X_i^\top \beta_0$ are independent and identically distributed before censoring. Assume the design variables X_i are bounded, and the error distribution satisfies*

$$\int_{-\infty}^{\infty} \frac{t^2}{1 - G(t-)} dF_\varepsilon(t) < \infty.$$

Then, as $n \to \infty$, we have

$$-2\log \frac{\sup_F EL_e(\beta_0, F)}{EL_e(\hat{\beta}, \hat{F}_{KM})} \longrightarrow \chi_p^2$$

in distribution, where $\hat{\beta}$ is the Buckley–James estimator, and both ELs are defined in (5.4) and the EL in the numerator is maximized under constraint (5.6).

The proof of this theorem is basically an application of the Wilks theorem for the mean constraints. We refer to Zhou and Li [142] for more details.

Example 21 *We illustrate the EL analysis of the Buckley–James estimator with the Stanford Heart Transplant data. Following Miller and Halpern [73], we use only 152 cases.*

```
library(survival)
data(stanford2)
stanford3 <- stanford2[!is.na(stanford2[,5]),]
stanford5 <- stanford3[(stanford3[,2]>=10),]
```

The specific AFT regression model we will fit is $\log_{10}(T_i) = \beta_1 + \beta_2 age + \varepsilon_i$. The following code tests $\beta_1 = 3.5, \beta_2 = -0.02$ and returns, among other things, the -2 log empirical likelihood ratio.

```
BJnoint(x=cbind(1,stanford5$age), y=log10(stanford5$time),
                delta=stanford5$status)
## $beta
## [1]   3.52749311 -0.01990791
##
## $iteration
## [1] 31
bjtest(y=log10(stanford5$time), d=stanford5$status,
          x=cbind(1,stanford5$age), beta=c(3.5, -0.02))
```

This test is repeated for many different values for the pair (β_1, β_2). The β pair values which lead to a (near) zero value of the -2 log likelihood ratio are the Buckley–James estimator. The collection of the values of the -2 log likelihood ratio corresponding to the different pairs of βs produces the contour plot in Fig. 5.1.

In the plot, the largest contour line is at level 5.99, making it the 95% confidence region for β_1, β_2 jointly. From the plot we see that the estimator $\hat{\beta}_1$ is negatively correlated with $\hat{\beta}_2$, since the contours point from upper left to the lower right. The 95% confidence interval for β_2 alone is approximately $[-0.036, -0.0026]$ and the 95% confidence interval for β_1 alone is approximately $[2.75, 4.25]$. These are obtained from the upper-left and lower-right points on the contour with level 3.84. They are approximate values because we used coarse grid points to produce the contour plot, and hence interpolation was used in the plot. Another way to find the confidence interval for individual βs will be presented in Chapter 6, Example 25.

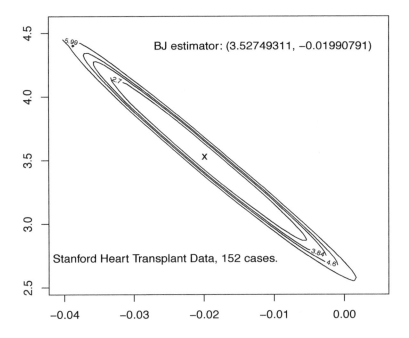

Figure 5.1: The -2 log empirical likelihood ratio contour plot, Stanford heart transplant data, 152 cases.

The center of the contours, marked by an X, is the Buckley–James estimator of β, the point where the -2 log likelihood ratio takes the the minimum value of zero. We can also infer from the plot that the contour lines are fairly close to a smooth ellipsoid, indicating that the normal approximation is quite reasonable for this example.

5.4 An Alternative EL Analysis for the Buckley–James Estimator

An alternative and simpler EL approach to the Buckley–James estimator also begins with the estimating equation (5.3), which we reproduce here:

$$0 = \sum_{j=1}^{n} \delta_j e_j(b) \left\{ X_j + \sum_{i:e_i<e_j,\delta_i=0} \frac{X_i \Delta \hat{F}(e_j)}{1-\hat{F}(e_i)} \right\}.$$

Without loss of generality, let us assume the terms in the above summation are always ordered according to the values of e_j. In other words, assume $e_1 < e_2 < \cdots < e_n$.

Suppose the hypothesis we are going to test is

$$H_0 : \beta = \beta_0 ,$$

against a two-sided alternative.

We further consider the situation where b takes the true value of the regression parameter, i.e., $b = \beta_0$. Under this assumption, the $(e_j(\beta_0), \delta_j)$ are the censored observations of the i.i.d. errors. More important, the curly bracket in (5.3) (as reproduced above) contains information at or before $e_j(\beta_0)$ but not after. This means the terms in the above sum depend on only $e_j(\beta_0)$, and predictable information at $e_j(\beta_0)$. Therefore, the summation in the above estimating equation can be viewed as a martingale integration against predictable functions and thus is a martingale itself.

Recall that we established a Wilks theorem for the EL of martingale differences (Theorem 2). Under the assumptions that the i.i.d. error ε_i have finite and positive variance, plus the boundedness of the design X_i, we can easily verify the regularity conditions for the M_j defined below; hence the following results hold.

Define the empirical likelihood function

$$EL = \prod_{i=1}^{n} p_i, \quad p_i \geq 0, \quad \sum p_i = 1 .$$

The test of the above null hypothesis can be based on

$$W = -2 \sup_{p_j} \left\{ \sum_{j=1}^{n} \log(p_j n) \mid p_j \geq 0; \ \sum p_j = 1 \text{ and } \sum p_j M_j = 0 \right\}$$

where

$$M_j = \delta_j e_j(\beta_0) \left\{ X_j + \sum_{i:e_i < e_j, \delta_i = 0} \frac{X_i \Delta \hat{F}(e_j)}{1 - \hat{F}(e_i)} \right\} .$$

By the Wilks theorem for martingale differences, the asymptotic distribution of W under H_0 is chi square with p degrees of freedom. Here $p = dim(\beta)$. We reject $H_0 : \beta = \beta_0$ if the value of W is larger than C. The threshold C can be determined by the chi square quantile with p degrees of freedom.

The computation of the log empirical likelihood ratio is particularly simple here because we can use the existing R function for the i.i.d. random vectors.

Zhu [144] ran some simulations comparing the null distribution of this empirical likelihood ratio with the empirical likelihood ratio of Section 5.3. For the examples she considered, the null distributions of the two log empirical likelihood ratios are similar to each other (both close to chi square). The confidence regions are also similar.

We illustrate this alternative EL test for the Buckley–James estimator using the Stanford Heart Transplant data.

The data `stanford5` was created in a previous example. Again, we test the hypothesis $\beta_1 = 3.5, \beta_2 = -0.02$ in the model

$$\log_{10}(\text{time}) = \beta_1 + \beta_2 \text{age} + \varepsilon .$$

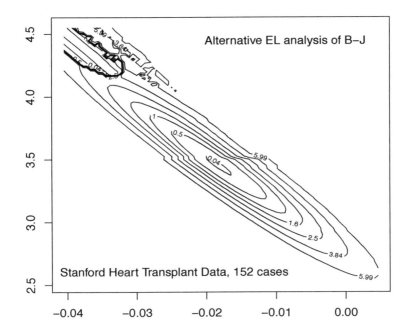

Figure 5.2: Alternative EL analysis of B–J. Contours of $-2 \log$ EL ratio. Compare to Fig. 5.1. Stanford heart transplant data, 152 cases.

This code runs faster than `bjtest( )`. For a single test this may not matter much. But for the computations to create a contour plot similar to Fig. 5.1, for profiling the empirical likelihood to get individual confidence intervals, this is appreciated. The two contour plots are somewhat similar. However, for the second plot (alternative EL analysis), the contour is less smooth and region is a bit wider. The second plot also exhibits chaotic behavior in the top region. We point out that Currie [17] also reported the chaotic behavior of the Buckley–James estimator. Whether the smoothness of contour can be improved with some smoothing modification on the martingale estimating equation (5.3) is an interesting question.

```
bjtestII(y=log10(stanford5$time), d=stanford5$status,
            x=cbind(1,stanford5$age), beta=c(3.5, -0.02))
## $'-2LLR'
## [1] 0.04997901
##
## $Pval
```

```
## [1] 0.9753201
## ......
```

5.5   Rank Estimator for the AFT Regression Model

We discussed the rank estimating equation for an AFT model in Chapter 2. We make a few remarks here.

(1) The AFT model we considered in Chapter 2 is what we called the AFT regression model, since the estimating equation is justified by i.i.d. errors via the residuals.

(2) We used the hazard formulation of the empirical likelihood in Chapter 2 with the rank estimating equations. By formulating similar constraints with respect to rank estimating equations, Zhou [137] proposed that the same *residual-wise* EL (defined in this chapter) be used with log rank or Gehan-type estimating equations. The resulting likelihood ratio admits a chi squared limiting distribution under the null hypothesis (Zhou [137]).

In fact, these two EL approaches yield nearly identical -2 log empirical likelihood ratios, thus producing the same estimators and confidence intervals (see the two programs below). However, the computation using the hazard EL of Chapter 2 is faster. Presumably, this is because the EL computation with CDFs is achieved via a slower EM algorithm.

Further comparison of these two empirical likelihood tests seems warranted. But the hazard formulation seems simpler and our R code is also faster.

```
library(emplik)
data(myeloma)
RankRegTest(y=log(myeloma[,1]), d=myeloma[,2],
                   x=myeloma[,3], beta=-2, type="Gehan")
RankRegTestH(y=log(myeloma[,1]), d=myeloma[,2],
                   x=myeloma[,3], beta=-2, type="Gehan")
```

5.6   AFT Correlation Models

The correlation model is appropriate if, for example, the goal is to estimate the regression plane for a certain population on the basis of a simple random sample (Freedman [29]). The true value of the parameter β solves

$$\int\int (y - x^\top \beta) x \, dF_{xy} = 0,$$

where F_{xy} denotes the joint $(p+1)$-variate distribution of x and y. Here, we assume that the vectors $(X_i, Y_i), i = 1, 2, \cdots, n$ are independent, the $p \times p$ covariance matrix of the rows of X, $EX^\top X$, is positive definite, and $E||(X,Y)||^3$ exists.

The estimation method we shall consider for this model is defined by the (case-wise weighted) estimating equation below. Weighted least squares and M-estimation methods have been proposed by Koul et al. [63], Zhou [135], Stute [108], and Gross and Lai [37]. The estimator b can be expressed as the solution of the estimating equations

$$\sum_{i=1}^{n} w_i(Z_i - X_i^{\top} b)X_i = 0, \tag{5.7}$$

with the weights w_i specified later in (5.9).

We note that this case-weighted estimator is very different from the "synthetic data" approach of Koul et al. [62], and Leurgans [66]. The "case-wise weighted" approach never creates any new response values (i.e., synthetic data). Instead, it tries to recoup the effect of censored responses by properly weighting the uncensored responses (in fact, this is how the Kaplan–Meier estimator works). On the other hand, it does not require iteration in the calculation of the estimator, as opposed to the Buckley–James estimator.

Two different weighting schemes are known in the literature to determine the weights w_i in Equation (5.7). Zhou [135] suggests using the jumps size of the Kaplan–Meier estimator computed on (Z_i, δ_i), as the weights. Stute [107] ordered the Z_i such that $\delta_{(i)}$ is the censoring indicator δ corresponding to the ith order statistic $Z_{(i)}$, and rewrote the jumps of the Kaplan–Meier estimator of the marginal distribution of Y as

$$\Delta_1 = \delta_{(1)}/n \quad \text{and} \quad \Delta_i = \frac{\delta_{(1)}}{n-i+1} \prod_{j=1}^{i-1} \left(\frac{n-j}{n-j+1}\right)^{\delta_{(j)}}, i = 2, \cdots, n. \tag{5.8}$$

He used the Δ_i as weights, w_i, in (5.7).

On the other hand, inverse probability-of-censoring weights have been used in many different places, for example, in van der Laan and Robins [119], Satten and Datta [99] and Rotnitzky and Robins [98]. The weights there are given by

$$w_i^* = \frac{\delta_i}{1 - \hat{G}(Z_i)} \tag{5.9}$$

with $\hat{G}(\cdot)$ being the Kaplan–Meier estimator of the censoring distribution G based on $(Z_i, 1 - \delta_i)$.

Inverse probability-of-censoring weighting is in fact equivalent to weighting by the jumps of the Kaplan–Meier estimator. Indeed, for all t,

$$[1 - \hat{F}(t)][1 - \hat{G}(t)] = 1 - \hat{H}(t) \tag{5.10}$$

where $\hat{F}(t)$ and $\hat{G}(t)$ are the Kaplan–Meier estimators for the distribution of Y_i based on (Z_i, δ_i) and the Kaplan–Meier estimator for the distribution of censoring variable C_i based on $(Z_i, 1 - \delta_i)$, respectively; $\hat{H}(t)$ is the empirical distribution based on Z_i. From (5.10), we may calculate the jump of each side when $t = Z_i$ with $\delta_i = 1$. This leads to $\Delta_i[1 - \hat{G}(t)] = 1/n$, from which it follows that

$$\Delta_i = \frac{\delta_i}{n[1 - \hat{G}(Z_i)]} = \frac{w_i^*}{n}. \tag{5.11}$$

Therefore the two weighting scheme produce the same weights.

Also, Stute [106] proposed using

$$\hat{F}_{xy}(A) = \sum_{i=1}^{n} \Delta_i I_{\{(Z_i, X_i) \in A\}} \quad \text{for set } A \text{ in } R^{(p+1)} \tag{5.12}$$

as a multivariate extension of the univariate Kaplan–Meier estimator. Based on these two observations, we call a solution to (5.7) with $w_i = \Delta_i$ a *case-wise* weighted estimator.

5.7   EL Analysis of AFT Correlation Models

Here we define the *case-wise* empirical likelihood for the AFT correlation model. Since (X_i, Y_i) are independent and identically distributed vectors (although Y_i are subject to censoring), we propose formulating the empirical likelihood *case-wise* as follows.

Consider the estimating equation $\int \int (y - x^\top \beta) x \, dF_{xy} = 0$. For any integrable function $\phi(x, y)$, equality holds for the two integrals

$$\int \int \phi(x, y) dF_{xy} \quad \text{and} \quad \int \int \phi(x, y) dF_{x|y} dF_y, \tag{5.13}$$

where $F_{x|y}$ denotes the conditional distribution of X given Y. Based on the data (X_i, Z_i, δ_i) $i = 1, \cdots n$, a reasonable estimator of $F_{x|y}$ when $y = Z_i$ and $\delta_i = 1$ is a point mass at X_i, because X_i is the one and only observation that satisfies $Z_i = y$ (assume Y has a continuous marginal distribution). In fact, using this conditional distribution coupled with the marginal distribution estimator $\hat{F}_y$, namely, the Kaplan–Meier estimator, one obtains an estimator that is identical to Stute's $\hat{F}_{xy}$ mentioned in (5.12) above.

Using this relationship, the *case-wise* empirical likelihood is

$$L_{xy}(F_y, F_{x|y}) = \prod 1 \prod_{\delta_i=1} p_i \prod_{\delta_i=0} \left(1 - \sum_{Z_j \leq Z_i} p_j\right), \tag{5.14}$$

where the $\prod 1$ is for $F(x|y)$, and $p_i = dF_y[Z_i]$ is the probability that F_y places on the ith case. Since the conditional distribution $F_{x|y}$ remains as a point mass throughout (as discussed above), we will from now on drop $F_{x|y}$ from L_{xy} and denote F_y simply as F. Similarly, we drop the constant point mass from the likelihood and finally get

$$L_{xy}(F_y) = \prod_{\delta_i=1} p_i \prod_{\delta_i=0} \left(1 - \sum_{Z_j \leq Z_i} p_j\right). \tag{5.15}$$

We want to emphasize that here $p_i = P(Y = Z_i)$.

The likelihood ratio is

$$R_{xy}(b) = \frac{\sup\{L_{xy}(F) | F \in \tilde{\mathbb{F}}^b\}}{\sup\{L_{xy}(F) | F \in \mathfrak{F}\}}, \tag{5.16}$$

where $\mathfrak{F}$ denotes the set of univariate distributions that place positive probabilities on each uncensored case (as $L_{xy}(F) = 0$ for any F that places zero probability on some uncensored (Z_i, δ_i)), and $\bar{\mathbb{F}}^b$ denotes a subset of $\mathfrak{F}$ that satisfies the constraints

$$\sum_{i=1}^{n} p_i \delta_i (Z_i - X_i^\top b) X_i = 0. \tag{5.17}$$

The above constraint is derived from (5.13) with (1) $\phi(x,y) = (y - x^\top \beta)x$, (2) a discrete $\hat{F}_y$ and (3) a point mass $\hat{F}_{x|y}$. It can also be interpreted as

$$\sum_{Z_i} \sum_{X_j} p_i \delta_i (Z_i - X_j^\top b) X_j d_{ij} = 0 \quad \text{or} \quad \int \int (y - x^\top b) x d\hat{F}_{xy} = 0$$

where $d_{ij} = 1$ if and only if $i = j$, and zero otherwise (reflecting $\hat{F}_{x|y}$), and $\hat{F}_{xy}$ is similar to Stute's estimator except we take $p_i = \Delta_i$.

It is easy to see that the maximum in the denominator of (5.16) occurs when F is the Kaplan–Meier estimator; hence the maximization calculation is required for the numerator only. The maximum can be obtained using the el.cen.EM2( ) function from the emplik package. When b is the *case-wise* weighted estimator (the solution to estimating equation (5.7)), then obviously the empirical likelihood ratio $R_{xy}(b) = 1$ and thus the confidence regions based on (5.16) are "centered" at this case-wise estimator.

Consider the AFT correlation model (5.1) with estimating equation (5.7). For testing the hypothesis $H_0 : \beta = \beta_0$ vs. $H_1 : \beta \neq \beta_0$, the following theorem contains the main result for the proposed *case-wise* empirical likelihood ratio statistic for least squares regression. A proof can be found in Zhou et al. [141].

Theorem 40 *Consider the AFT correlation model as specified above. Under H_0 : $\beta = \beta_0$ and assuming regularity conditions (C1)–(C3) and (C6) specified below, $-2 \log R_{xy}(\beta_0) \to \chi_p^2$ in distribution as $n \to \infty$.*

Regularity conditions.
(C1) The (transformed) survival times Y_i and the censoring times C_i are independent. Furthermore, $P(Y_i \leq C_i | X_i, Y_i) = P(Y_i \leq C_i | Y_i)$.
(C2) The survival functions $P(Y_i \geq t)$ and $P(C_i \geq t)$ are continuous and either $\xi_Y < \xi_C$ or $\forall t < \infty, P(Z_i \geq t) > 0$. Here, for any random variable U, ξ_U denotes the right end point of the support of U.
(C3) The X_i are independent, identically distributed according to some distribution with finite, nonzero variance, and they are independent of Y_i and C_i.
(C4) $0 < \sigma_{KM}^2(\phi) < \infty$ where $\sigma_{KM}^2(\phi)$ is the asymptotic variance of $\sqrt{n} \Sigma_i (t_i - x_i^\top \beta) x_i \Delta \hat{F}_{KM}(t_i)$.

In many applications, inference is sought for only part of the β parameter vector. A typical approach is to "profile" out the parameters that are not under consideration.

Profiling has been proposed for empirical likelihood in uncensored cases (e.g., Qin and Lawless [92]). Under censoring, Lin and Wei [70] proposed profiling with Buckley–James estimators. We similarly consider a profile empirical likelihood ratio:

let $\beta = (\beta_1, \beta_2)$ where $\beta_1 \in R^q$ with $q < p$ is the part of the parameter under testing. Similarly, let $\beta_0 = (\beta_{10}, \beta_{20})$. A profile empirical likelihood ratio for β_1 is given by

$$\sup_{\beta_2} R_{xy}(\beta = (\beta_1, \beta_2)) .$$

The theorem below states that Wilks theorem holds for the profile empirical likelihood as well.

Theorem 41 *Consider the AFT correlation model as specified above. Suppose the parameter vector has been divided into two parts:* $\beta = (\beta_1, \beta_2)$. *Assume the same conditions of Theorem 40 above. Under the composite hypothesis* $H_0 : \beta_1 = \beta_{10}$, *we have* $-2\log \sup_{\beta_2} R_{xy}(\beta = (\beta_{10}, \beta_2)) \to\Rightarrow \chi_q^2$ *in distribution as* $n \to \infty$, *where* $q = dim(\beta_1)$.

Computation of profiling may not be easy, especially when the β dimension is larger than 5, for example. Examples of profiling an empirical likelihood can be found in Chapter 6.

We include below some code that (1) simulates data from an AFT model $Y = x + \varepsilon$, (2) calculate the (case weighted) estimator, and (3) use case-wise EL to find the 95% confidence interval for the regression parameter (true value of the parameter $= 1$).

```
Simulat <- function(N=90, mu=3) {
x <- rnorm(N, mean=1, sd=0.5)
eps <- rnorm(N, sd=0.5)
y <- x + eps
cen <- rnorm(N, mean=mu, sd=4)
ycen <- pmin(cen, y)
d <- as.numeric( y <= cen )

out1 <- WRegEst(x=x, y=ycen, delta=d)
out2 <- WRegTest(x=x, y=ycen, delta=d, beta0=1)

myfunUL <- function(theta, x, y, d){
            WRegTest(x=x, y=y, delta=d, beta0=theta)
}
out3 <- findUL(fun=myfunUL, MLE=out1, x=x, y=ycen, d=d)

list(Est=out1, "-2LLR"=out2$"-2LLR",
                          ConInt=c(out3$Low, out3$Up) )
}
```

5.7.1 Quantile Regression Models

Similar results (Theorems 40 and 41) hold for censored quantile regression models when the τth conditional quantile of Y_i is modeled by

$$Q_\tau(\log T_i|X_i) = Q_\tau(Y_i|X_i) = X_i^\top \beta_\tau,$$

and, instead of $Y_i = \log T_i$, we observe $Z_i = \min(Y_i, C_i)$ and $\delta_i = I_{[Y_i \leq C_i]}$ for some censoring time variables C_i. This model may also be written as $Y_i = X_i^\top \beta_\tau + e_i$, where the error terms e_i are just independent random variables with zero τth quantile. When $\tau = 0.5$, this is the censored median regression, and Huang et al. [45] proposed a *case-wise* weighted estimator, which is a special case of our *case-wise* weighted estimator. Here, we propose the following *case-wise* empirical likelihood inference for the general censored quantile regression using

$$\mathbb{R}_{xy}(b) = \frac{\sup\{L_{xy}(F)|F \in \tilde{\mathbb{F}}^b\}}{\sup\{L_{xy}(F)|F \in \mathfrak{F}\}}, \tag{5.18}$$

where $\tilde{\mathbb{F}}^b$ denotes a subset of $\mathfrak{F}$ that satisfies the constraints

$$\sum_{i=1}^n p_i \delta_i \psi_\tau(Z_i - X_i^\top b)X_i = 0, \tag{5.19}$$

and $\psi_\tau(u)$ is the derivative of the so-called check function $\rho_\tau(u) = u(\tau - I_{[u<0]})$ of Koenker and Basset [61]. Similar to the censored accelerated failure time model, the denominator of $\mathbb{R}_{xy}(b)$ is maximized by the Kaplan–Meier estimator, and thus when calculating $\mathbb{R}_{xy}(b)$ the maximization is only needed for the numerator.

Theorem 42 *Assume regularity conditions (C1)–(C3) of Theorem 40 above plus two more conditions (C5), (C6) below hold. Under $H_0 : \beta_\tau = \beta_0$, for given τ, $-2\log \mathbb{R}_{xy}(\beta_0) \to \chi_p^2$ in distribution as $n \to \infty$. If $\beta_\tau = (\beta_1, \beta_2)$ with $\beta_1 \in R^q$ with $q < p$, under $H_0 : \beta_1 = \beta_{10}$, we have $-2\log \sup_{\beta_2} \mathbb{R}_{xy}(\beta_\tau = (\beta_{10}, \beta_2)) \to \chi_q^2$ in distribution as $n \to \infty$.*

(C5) Let $F_e(\cdot|x)$ be the conditional distribution of e_i given $X = x$, and $f_e(\cdot|x)$ be the corresponding conditional density function. For the given τ, $F_e(0|x) = \tau$, and $f_e(u|x)$ is continuous in u in a neighborhood of 0 for almost all x.
(C6) $E(XX^\top f_e(0|X))$ is finite and nonsingular.

Example 22 *We illustrate how to obtain a p-value in a testing hypothesis set-up within a censored quantile regression model. We consider a lung cancer dataset that has been analyzed by Ying et al. [131] using median regression, and by Huang et al. [45] using a least absolute deviation method in the AFT model.*

In this study, 121 patients with limited-stage small-cell lung cancer were randomly assigned to one of two different treatment sequences A and B, with 62 patients assigned to A and 59 patients to B. Each death time was either observed or administratively censored, and the censoring variable did not depend on the covariates treatment *and* age.

Denote the treatment indicator variable by X_{1i}, and the entry age for the ith patient by X_{2i}, where $X_{1i} = 1$ if the patient is in group B. Let Y_i be the base 10 logarithm of the ith patient's failure time. We assume the AFT model

$$Y_i = \beta_1 + \beta_2 X_{1i} + \beta_3 X_{2i} + \sigma(X_{1i}, X_{2i})\varepsilon_i .$$

The following median regression estimates were obtained by Huang et al. [45].

$$\hat{\beta}_1 = 2.693, \ \hat{\beta}_2 = -0.146, \ and \ \hat{\beta}_3 = 0.001 . \tag{5.20}$$

Huang et al. [45] did not always treat the largest Z observation $(Z = \min(Y,C))$ as uncensored. This resulted in weights that sum to less than one in this dataset (the sum of the weights without the last observation is 0.85). We recommend treating the largest Z observation as uncensored so that the weights always sum to one. Otherwise, the estimation may be biased since the information from the largest Z observation is ignored. Treating the largest Z as uncensored, the case-weight median regression estimates become

$$\hat{\beta}_1 = 2.603, \ \hat{\beta}_2 = -0.263, \ and \ \hat{\beta}_3 = 0.0038 \quad \textit{(with last weight)}. \tag{5.21}$$

```
library(emplik)
data(smallcell)
Z <- log10(smallcell$survival)
dd <- smallcell$indicator
temp <- WKM(x=Z, d=dd, zc=1:121)
KMweight2 <- temp$jump
sum(KMweight2)
## [1] 1

norder <- order(smallcell$survival)
temp2 <- rq.wfit(x=cbind(1, smallcell$arm[norder],
                   smallcell$entry[norder]),
                y=Z[norder], weights=KMweight2)
coef(temp2)
## [1]   2.603342985 -0.263000044   0.003836832

myfunq <- function(y, xmat) {
    mytemp1 <- as.vector(y -(2.6+xmat %*% c(-0.263,0.004)))
    mytemp2 <- as.numeric(mytemp1 > 0) +
                   as.numeric(mytemp1 >= 0) - 1
    return(cbind(mytemp2, mytemp2*xmat))
    }
XX <- cbind(smallcell$arm, smallcell$entry)
temp3 <- el.cen.EM2(x=Z, d=dd, fun=myfunq,
                   mu=c(0,0,0), xmat=XX)
temp3$"-2LLR"
## [1] 0.1473368
```

The p-value of this log empirical likelihood ratio should be computed using a chi square distribution with three degrees of freedom. We leave this to the reader.

In a simulation study Zhou et al. [141] compared the confidence intervals obtained from empirical likelihood to those obtained by bootstrap (see Huang et al. [45]). They found that two types of confidence intervals behave very similarly in length and coverage probability, with the EL interval slightly less varied.

5.8 Discussion and Historical Remarks

BUCKLEY–JAMES ESTIMATOR

The Buckley–James estimator was proposed in 1979 and found to be competitive with the Cox regression model, particularly for predicting purposes in several studies. See Miller and Halpern [73] and Heller and Simonoff [39]. However, the use of the Buckley–James estimator and AFT models in practice is still limited. Part of the reason is the extraordinary success of the Cox regression model.

Also, there is no easy way to calculate the variance of the Buckley–James estimator, hence the confidence interval and *p*-value are hard to compute. In addition, the iterative algorithm for solving the Buckley–James estimation equation may not converge, and sometimes has chaotic behavior. Smoothing has been proposed as a possible way to alleviate the chaotic behavior but so far there has been limited success.

The large sample properties of the Buckley–James estimator have been investigated by Lai and Ying [64]. In particular, they pointed out that the variance estimation formula proposed by Buckley and James is not consistent. This fact has been confirmed by Zhou and Li [142] in simulations. It is found that the original formula, as implemented by the bj( ) function of the R rms library, gives *p*-values that are too conservative.

The treatment of the Buckley–James estimator EL analysis presented here is based on Zhou and Li [142]. In a 2007 University of Kentucky Ph.D. dissertation [144], Zhu studied several variations and extensions of the Zhou and Li [142] EL treatment for the Buckley–James estimator. Some of the variations are simpler to calculate and still yield a chi square distribution under the null hypothesis for the log EL ratio. More studies of the different EL approaches to the Buckley–James estimator are needed in order to decide which approach is preferred.

QUANTILE REGRESSION

Quantile regression was discussed in Koenker [60]. With random right censored data, median regression was studied by Ying et al. [131]. The variance of the estimators can be difficult to obtain, since it involves the density of an unknown distribution. For the regression estimator proposed by Ying et al. [131], its variance estimation requires the inversion of an estimated variance-covariance matrix, which may be unstable, particularly at the tails of the survival functions.

Portnoy [87] investigated the censored quantile regression process using a recursive algorithm that fits the *entire* quantile regression process successively from below. His method, however, requires the strong assumption that the entire qunatile process is linear in x_i. Thus the validity of quantile estimates at, for example, the median depends on the linearity of all conditional functionals at all lower quantiles; nonlinear relations at any of the lower quantiles will bias the median estimates.

Note that the estimated parameter values we obtained using the approach described here are the same as those from Huang et al. [45], provided the weighting of the last observation is done in the same way. The major difference is in the inference about the parameters, where empirical likelihood has the advantage that it is not necessary to estimate the asymptotic variance of the estimator in order to perform hypothesis tests and to construct confidence regions.

RANK-BASED ESTIMATORS

One difficulty with the rank estimating equation and censored data is that the solution of the equations can be tricky to obtain. Without censoring, the estimating function is monotone in β. With censoring, Fygenson and Ritov [30] showed that the Gehan estimating function is also monotone. However, in an effort to achieve efficiency, other weights are needed. The log rank estimating function does not result in monotone estimating functions. To make things worse, the estimating function is not continuous. Heller [38] tried to smooth the functions to achieve continuity.

For rank estimator with Gehan weights, we can use the R package lss or aftgee to compute the estimator.

5.9   Exercise

Exercise 5.1 *Use the dataset* smallcell *from the package* emplik. *Fit an AFT correlation model using treatment and age at entry as two covariates.*

Chapter 6

Computation of Empirical Likelihood Ratio with Censored Data

The computation of the empirical likelihood ratio is closely related to the computation of the nonparametric maximum likelihood estimators (NPMLE) and the *constrained* NPMLE. For right censored data, the NPMLE of the CDF is the Kaplan–Meier estimator and the NPMLE of the cumulative hazard function is the Nelson–Aalen estimator, which are both explicitly given and easy to compute. The constrained versions do not have an explicit formula and are harder to calculate. We discuss in this chapter several methods and the related issues in computing the constrained Kaplan–Meier and Nelson–Aalen estimators and the related empirical likelihood ratios. The methods include the Newton type iteration, Lagrange multiplier technique and expectation-maximization (EM) algorithm. Their implementation in R is also discussed.

6.1 Empirical Likelihood for Uncensored Data

The theory for the empirical likelihood ratio test for uncensored data was developed by Owen and can be found in his book [81]. We formulated a version of the key Wilks theorem in Chapter 1 as Theorem 1. There are also many refinements of this theorem, some of which can be found in the reference list of Owen's book.

The R package emplik includes a function el.test( ) for calculating the empirical likelihood ratio in this uncensored data case. The available data are assumed to be n i.i.d. random vectors of dimension p:

$$\mathbf{X}_i = (X_{i1}, X_{i2}, \cdots, X_{ip}) \quad \text{for } i = 1, 2, \cdots, n.$$

The log empirical likelihood function is assumed to be

$$\log EL = \sum_{i=1}^{n} \log w_i \quad \text{with } \sum_{i=1}^{n} w_i = 1$$

where $w_i = P(\mathbf{X}_i)$.

The null hypothesis we are testing is specified as

$$H_0 : EX_{11} = \mu_1, EX_{12} = \mu_2, \cdots, EX_{1p} = \mu_p. \tag{6.1}$$

137

Without the p constraints of H_0, the NPMLE of the CDF is the empirical distribution: a CDF that puts $w_i = 1/n$ at each observed $\mathbf{X}_i$. This leads to the maximum value of the EL: $\prod(1/n) = (1/n)^n$. The constrained NPMLE in this case is the tilted empirical distribution with

$$w_i(\lambda) = \frac{1}{n - \lambda^\top(\mathbf{X}_i - \mu)}.$$

The amount of tilting, controlled by λ, is to satisfy the p constraint equations specified in H_0. To find the exact amount of tilting, we need to solve the following p equations for λ:

$$\sum_{i=1}^{n} \frac{X_{ik} - \mu_k}{n - \lambda^\top(\mathbf{X}_i - \mu)} = 0 \quad \text{for } k = 1, 2, \cdots, p. \tag{6.2}$$

The R function el.test( ) uses the damped Newton iteration method to solve the p equations (6.2), and then returns the empirical likelihood ratio as well as those $w_i(\lambda)$'s.

If instead the null hypothesis is

$$H_0 : Eg_1(X_1) = \mu_1, \cdots, Eg_p(X_p) = \mu_p,$$

then we need to first apply the g transformation to the original data, and then input the transformed data into el.test( ):

$$(g_1(X_{i1}), \cdots, g_p(X_{ip})) \quad i = 1, 2, \cdots, n$$

and then call the function el.test( ).

In the function el.test( ), the dimension of the input data $X_i\ i = 1, 2, \cdots, n$, is always assumed to be equal to the number of mean constraints.

The package emplik also includes a weighted version of the above empirical likelihood ratio test: el.test.wt2( ). This is designed to solve the following problems: We assume, in addition to the n independent observations X_i, there is a given, fixed, nonnegative weight vector, $v_1, v_2, \cdots, v_n$. Also, we work with a weighted log empirical likelihood function

$$\log EL = \sum_{i=1}^{n} v_i \log w_i, \quad \text{with } w_i \geq 0; \ \sum_{i=1}^{n} w_i = 1. \tag{6.3}$$

The hypothesis to be tested is the same as (6.1), which in vector form is

$$H_0 : \sum_{i=1}^{n} w_i \mathbf{X}_i = \mu.$$

Obviously, when all the weights $v_i = 1$, this is the same as the el.test( ). But in some applications we may want to set v_i to something else. This function was originally an internal function written for use with the EM algorithm calculation of the constrained Kaplan–Meier estimator, but it was found to be useful in various other applications of empirical likelihood; see, for example, Chapter 7. So it became a stand-alone function.

Recently, Yang and Small [128] and Owen [82] investigated an alternative to the computational algorithm used in el.test( ). The potential problem for the el.test( ) seems to be when the constraint is a vector of means, and the constrained mean values for the CDF (6.1) are nearly impossible. This corresponds to the case when the constraint values μ are near the boundary of the convex hull of the observed data. In terms of confidence regions, this corresponds to the case when we try to compute a confidence region with a very high nominal confidence level (of 0.9999999 or above). In terms of a test, this corresponds to the cases when the p-values are 0.0000001 or smaller. This confidence level is seldom used in practice. If this cannot be avoided, Yang and Small recommend that researchers who want to find the empirical likelihood should consider the el.test( ) first, and check the condition whether the weights (probabilities) sum to one. If they do not, one should use the R package el.convex or function scel.R from Owen's web page instead.

When the number of constraints exceeds the number of parameters (dimension of input X), i.e., the over-determined estimating equation case, there is the R package gmm. It includes an empirical likelihood solution to those estimating problems alongside the generalized method of moments, from which the package got its name. However, there does not seem to be a similar function in R for right censored data yet.

6.2   EL after Jackknife

Under mild conditions, the empirical likelihood ratio test statistic has a null distribution of chi square (Chapter 1, Theorem 1). One of the conditions necessary for the uncensored data EL Theorem 1 to hold is that the observations X_i are (asymptotically) i.i.d. and the statistic of interest is the sample mean or sum. Sometimes the original data/statistics do not satisfy this requirement, but can be approximated by an i.i.d. mean after some transformation.

One such case is provided by the jackknife pseudo values of a U-statistic (Jing et al. [49]).

Example 23 *(Jackknife empirical likelihood) Let $X_1, X_2, \cdots, X_n$ be i.i.d. random variables. Suppose $h(x,y)$ is a function that is symmetric in its two arguments. In addition, we assume the mean $Eh(X_1, X_2)$ is well-defined, and the variance of $h(X_1, X_2)$ is finite and positive.*

Define the (one sample, order 2) U-statistic

$$U_n = \frac{1}{n(n-1)} \sum_{1 \leq i < j \leq n} h(X_i, X_j) . \qquad (6.4)$$

This is an unbiased estimator of the mean $Eh(X_1, X_2)$, but the terms in the U_n summation are obviously dependent, for example, due to the fact that $h(X_1, X_2)$ and $h(X_2, X_3)$ share a common variable X_2.

Jing et al. [49] suggest that we define jackknife pseudo values V_{nj} and then apply the (uncensored data) empirical likelihood method to those pseudo values

$$V_{nj} = nU_n - (n-1)U_{n-1}^{-j}, \quad j = 1, 2, \cdots, n, \tag{6.5}$$

where U_{n-1}^{-j} denotes the U-statistic based on the $n-1$ observations: all the X_i's except X_j. It turns out that these pseudo values are often asymptotically independent and have mean approximately equal to $Eh(X_1, X_2)$; thus Owen's empirical likelihood ratio theorem (Theorem 1) applies to the test of the mean of those pseudo values.

Let us take $h(x, y) = |x - y|$ and test the hypothesis

$$H_0 : E|X_1 - X_2| = \mu .$$

```
library(bootstrap)
library(emplik)
set.seed(123)
xsample <- rexp(100)
thetafun <- function(x) {
            N <- length(x)
            hfun <- function(x,y){abs(x-y)}
            A <- outer(x, x, FUN= hfun)
            temp <- sum( A[upper.tri(A)] )
            return( temp/(N*(N-1)) )
}
jackX <- jackknife(x=xsample, theta=thetafun)$jack.values
pseudoX <- 100*thetafun(xsample) - 99*jackX
el.test(x=pseudoX, mu=0.5)
## $'-2LLR'
## [1] 0.009114737
##
## $Pval
## [1] 0.9239406
## ......
```

We can also obtain the confidence interval of the parameter $E|X_1 - X_2|$ by invert- ing the empirical likelihood ratio test.

```
myfun8 <- function(theta, x) {
        el.test(x=x, mu=theta)
        }
findUL(fun=myfun8, MLE=0.5, x=pseudoX)
## $Low
## [1] 0.3972289
##
## $Up
## [1] 0.6867303
## ...
```

We see the asymptotic 95% confidence interval is $[0.3972289, 0.6867303]$.

We want to point out that using the i.i.d. sum to approximate the U-statistic is very similar to the idea of Hoeffding projection approximation. In other words, find the function $g_n(X_i)$ *as a projection of* U_n *in an* L_2 *space, and show that*

$$U_n - \frac{1}{n} \sum_{i=1}^{n} g_n(X_i) = o_p(\frac{1}{\sqrt{n}}) \ .$$

We then switch the problem of testing the mean of U_n *or* $h(X_1, X_2)$ *to testing the mean of* $g_n(X_1)$, *by using the sample mean* $\sum g_n(X_i)/n$. *Since the terms in this summation,* $g_n(X_i)$, *are i.i.d., the original empirical likelihood ratio theorem of Owen applies.*

Our next example deals with the statistic of the Kaplan–Meier estimator. It also illustrates that before we compute the jackknife pseudo values, it often helps to apply a transformation to the statistics of interest. In other words, we might jackknife the arcsine square root of the Kaplan–Meier survival probability estimator, as suggested by Gaver and Miller [33].

Gaver and Miller [33] investigated the use of jackknife with a Kaplan–Meier estimator and the construction of confidence intervals. Stute and Wang [109] only used the jackknife to estimate the bias. Stute [107] is concerned with the estimation of the variance of a Kaplan–Meier integral. But Gaver and Miller went further and used the jackknife to construct confidence intervals.

However, in their simulations, the resulting confidence intervals from the jackknife method tend toward overcoverage and perform no better than the EL-based confidence intervals. Their only criticism for the EL-based confidence interval is the computation cost. The high computational cost made them abandon the simulation for the case of sample size $n = 50$ for the EL-based confidence intervals. But that was in 1983. Now the computational burden for the EL-based confidence interval is not a problem. It takes about 80 seconds to complete 1000 EL confidence intervals for *all* time t on today's average laptop computer.

Example 24 *We shall carry out a simulation that Gaver and Miller [33] forfeited. We shall also try the (uncensored data) EL after the jackknife pseudo values are obtained (as suggested by Jing et al. [49]). The simulation setup is: sample size* $n = 50$, *survival distribution is unit exponential, censoring distribution is uniform* $(0, 1)$ *and* $(0, 1.5)$. *The statistic of interest is the Kaplan–Meier estimator of survival probability at* t_0, *with* t_0 *chosen to have the true survival equal to 0.5.*

```
library(emplik)
library(survival)
library(km.ci)

theta6.2 <- function(x, d){
temp <- WKM(x=x,d=d)
indx <- sum(temp$times < log(2))
```

```
surv0.5 <- temp$surv[indx]
return( asin(sqrt(surv0.5)) )
}


Jpseudo <- function(x, d){
N <- length(x)
Jps <- rep(NA, N)
for( i in 1:N ) Jps[i] <- theta6.2(x=x[-i], d=d[-i])
return(N*theta6.2(x=x, d=d) - (N-1)*Jps)
}


SIMU6.2 <- function(N=50, maxi=1.5, t = -log(0.5)){
xvec <- rexp(N)
cvec <- runif(N, min=0, max=maxi)
yvec <- pmin(xvec, cvec)
dvec <- as.numeric( xvec <= cvec)

JSvec <- Jpseudo(x=yvec, d=dvec)
est <- theta6.2(x=yvec, d=dvec)
se <- sum((JSvec - mean(JSvec))^2)/(N-1)
se <- sqrt(se)
loo <- est - 1.96*se/sqrt(N)
upp <- est + 1.96*se/sqrt(N)
loo <- (sin(loo))^2
upp <- (sin(upp))^2

LLR <- el.test(x=JSvec, mu=asin(sqrt(0.5)))$"-2LLR"

sfit <- survfit(Surv(yvec, dvec)~1)
temp <- summary( km.ci(survi=sfit, method="grunkemeier") )
indx <- sum(temp$time < t)
lo <- temp$lower[indx]
up <- temp$upper[indx]
return(c(lo,up, loo, upp, LLR) )
}


set.seed(123)
SIMU6.2(maxi=1)        # just one simulation run
```

Using a censoring distribution of uniform $(0, 1)$ (implies a censoring percentage around 63%) and 50,000 simulation runs, we get:

• The nominal 95% confidence interval by the EL of Thomas and Grunkemeier has coverage probability $1 - 0.05598$.

• The transformation plus jackknife confidence interval has coverage probability $1 - 0.04622$.

• *The (uncensored) EL confidence interval based on the jackknife pseudo values has coverage probability* $1 - 0.02522$.

Using a censoring distribution of uniform $(0, 1.5)$ *(implies a censoring percentage around 52%), we get*
• *The nominal 95% confidence interval by EL of Thomas and Grunkemeier has coverage probability* $1 - 0.05062$.
• *The transformation plus jackknife confidence interval has coverage probability* $1 - 0.04656$.
• *The (uncensored) EL confidence interval based on the jackknife pseudo values has coverage probability* $1 - 0.03244$.

In this example, the (uncensored) EL after the jackknife pseudo values does not perform well (severe overcoverage). In addition, it also loses the "transformation invariant" property of the (censored) EL confidence interval.

Our recommendation is to use the Thomas and Grunkemeier EL directly with the original censored data.

Remark: For small samples the Thomas and Grunkemeier confidence interval may be slightly under cover. We may consider replace the chi square distribution with a distribution of student t-distribution square, $t^2(k)$, in the construction of confidence interval. The choice for the degree of freedom k for the t-distribution should depend on the actual sample size and the censoring rate.

6.3 One- or Two-Sample Hazard Features

The log empirical likelihood in terms of hazard was discussed in Chapter 1 and Chapter 2. The maximization of the hazard log empirical likelihood, with and without constraints, was also studied in Chapter 2. We recall the following facts:

(1) The unconstrained NPMLE of the cumulative hazard function is the so-called Nelson–Aalen estimator. It is explicitly given in (1.31) and is denoted by $\hat{\Lambda}_{NA}(t)$.

(2) For constraints that are specified by $\int g(t)d\Lambda(t) = \theta$, which works with the Poisson version of the censored log empirical likelihood (2.3), the constrained NPMLE of the cumulative hazard function (or its jumps) is given by

$$w_i(\lambda) = \frac{\delta_i \Delta \hat{\Lambda}_{NA}(T_i)}{1 + \lambda^\top Z_i}, \tag{6.6}$$

where $Z_i = \frac{\delta g(T_i)}{R_i/n}$ and λ controls the amount of tilting and is the solution of the equation

$$\frac{1}{n} \sum_{i=1}^{n-1} \frac{\delta_i Z_i}{1 + \lambda^\top Z_i} + \delta_n g(T_n) = \theta. \tag{6.7}$$

Since this corresponds to a purely discrete cumulative hazard function, the jumps must satisfy $w_i \in [0, 1)$, with the exception of the last jump. The last jump (at the largest T_i value) is either 0 when $\delta = 0$ or 1 when $\delta = 1$. These restrictions on w_i delimit the legitimate values of λ. We call these legitimate values the feasible values of λ. Therefore, every solution for λ needs to be checked for conformance of the w_i to these requirements.

Otherwise, either the θ value in the constraint (6.7) is too far away from the NPMLE (in this case, the -2 log likelihood ratio should be defined as infinity, indicating that no hazard satisfies the constraints), or the iterative method used to solve Equation (6.7) has a trial solution that is too aggressive. Although we try to minimize the possibility of the second situation, it does happen sometimes, especially when θ is near the boundary of the feasible values.

It is obvious that λ and θ are monotonically related via Equation (6.7) when λ belongs to its feasible region. We therefore shall call the θ value feasible when the corresponding λ values are feasible.

Also, obviously $\lambda = 0$ always belongs to the feasible set for λ, in which case the Nelson–Aalen estimator and its jumps automatically satisfy the requirement $w_i \in [0,1)$. The corresponding θ is $\int g(t)d\hat{\Lambda}_{NA}(t)$, which is the NPMLE of θ; thus the NPMLE of θ, denoted by $\hat{\theta}$, always belongs to the feasible set of θ.

These observations help us to compute the constrained NPMLE when it does exist, and to report error when the constrained θ is outside the feasible set.

The R package `emplik` contains several functions to compute empirical likelihood ratios for right censored data for the problem setup just described.

The functions `emplikH1.test( )` and `emplikH2.test( )` are for testing a single constraint of the form (explicit function or implicit function)

$$\int g(t)d\Lambda(t) = \theta$$

and

$$\int g(t,\theta)d\Lambda(t) = K .$$

The function `emplikHs.test2( )` can handle multiple constraints and two-sample test problems.

In the two-sample setup, we assume there are two independent samples, both subject to right censoring. The null hypothesis for this function `emplikHs.test2( )` is assumed to be specified by

$$H_0 : \int g_1(t)d\Lambda_1(t) - \int g_2(t)d\Lambda_2(t) = \theta ,$$

where both g_1, g_2 and θ can be multi-dimensional. But they must be of the same dimension.

Also, $\Lambda_1(t)$ above denotes the cumulative hazard of the sample one, and $\Lambda_2(t)$ denotes the cumulative hazard of the sample two.

If you have a one sample problem, with multiple constraints, you can still use this function. You just need to input some fake data as sample two, and define your $g_2()$ function as identically zero. The fake data can consist of a few observations or a few dozen observations. In the output, there is a likelihood for sample one only.

We give a series of examples that illustrate the capability of the function in the package `emplik`.

The above R functions all use the so-called Poisson version of the empirical like-lihood function. The `emplik` package also contains parallel functions which use bi-nomial empirical likelihood functions.

The function `emplikH.disc( )` is for computing the binomial empirical likeli-hood ratio with one sample of right censored observations, one parameter, and under the hypothesis specified as

$$H_0 : \sum_i f(t_i, \theta) \log[1 - d\Lambda(t_i)] = K .$$

On the other hand, `emplikH.disc2( )` is for computing the two-sample bino-mial empirical likelihood ratio and a one-dimensional parameter θ defined for two samples of right censored observations with a null hypothesis

$$H_0 : \sum_i f_1(t_i) \log[1 - d\Lambda_1(t_i)] - \sum_j f_2(t_j) \log[1 - d\Lambda_2(t_j)] = \theta .$$

The function `emplikHs.disc2( )` is for multiple parameters and two samples (similar to `emplikHs.test2( )` but using binomial empirical likelihood). The null hypothesis under consideration is

$$H_0 : \sum_i \mathbf{f}_1(t_i) \log[1 - d\Lambda_1(t_i)] - \sum_j \mathbf{f}_2(t_j) \log[1 - d\Lambda_2(t_j)] = \boldsymbol{\theta} ,$$

where $\mathbf{f}_1$, $\mathbf{f}_2$ and $\boldsymbol{\theta}$ can all be vectors but they must be of the same dimension.

If you want to compute the binomial empirical likelihood ratio for one sample, multiple parameters, you may still use `emplikHs.disc2( )`. Just define $\mathbf{f}_2$ as iden-tically zero and supplying some fake data as sample two, we then read the calculated -2 log likelihood ratio only for sample one.

6.4 Empirical Likelihood Testing Concerning Mean Functions

Unlike the hazard empirical likelihood, the constrained NPMLE for the mean case in Chapter 3 does not have an easy method of calculation.

As discussed in Chapter 1, the unconstrained maximization of the log empirical likelihood, $\log EL_1$ in (1.24), is achieved by the Kaplan–Meier estimator.

The maximized censored data empirical likelihood, under the mean constraints

$$\sum_{i=1}^{n} g(T_i) w_i = \mu ,$$

does not seem to have an explicit formula. One possible approach is to use traditional iterative methods: (1) a sequential quadratic programming method or (2) a modified EM algorithm to accommodate constraints.

The R package `emplik` provides both of these two computation methods for the constrained NPMLE and related empirical likelihood ratio. However, the sequential quadratic programming method can be very memory hungry for sample sizes over a few hundred. The EM algorithm is a lot better in the memory requirement, but may require a large number of iterations before convergence.

6.4.1   EM Algorithm

Here we briefly describe the EM algorithm in a generic manner. Suppose we are given censored data (T_i, δ_i), and a mean constraint equation for the CDF.

Step 0. (Initialization) Pick an initial (discrete) CDF F which may or may not satisfy the given mean constraint. The support of this CDF should be the entire uncensored observed times. We use the Kaplan–Meier estimator $\hat{F}_{KM}(\cdot)$ as the initial estimator (with possible modification of the last observation to guarantee a proper distribution).

Step 1. (E-step) Find the conditional probability with respect to F that an observation is equal to X_i, given the sample $(T_j, \delta_j), j = 1, 2, \cdots, n$. This step is the same as the E-step of Turnbull [118] and will produce pseudo observations X_i and weights w_i.

Step 2. (M-step) With the (X_i, w_i) from the E-step above, find a new CDF estimate F (or equivalently the $p_i = dF(X_i)$'s) using the formula

$$p_i = \frac{w_i}{\sum_j w_j + \lambda (g(X_i) - \mu)}, \tag{6.8}$$

where λ is the solution of the equation

$$\sum_i \frac{w_i (g(X_i) - \mu)}{\sum_j w_j + \lambda (g(X_i) - \mu)} = 0. \tag{6.9}$$

This new CDF will satisfy the mean constraint (null hypothesis).

Step 3. Iterate Steps 1 and 2 until convergence.

Zhou [138] showed that this iteration converges to the desired constrained maximization solution. Specifically, he showed that the solution of the EM algorithm is equivalent to the solution of constrained maximization of the log empirical likelihood. For details see the paper by Zhou [138].

This algorithm is implemented in the package `emplik` by the functions `el.cen.EM2( )` and `el.cen.EM( )`. The function `el.cen.EM( )` can only take one mean type constraint, but is faster. On the other hand, `el.cen.EM2( )` can handle multiple mean type constraints. As just pointed out, the EM algorithm can be a bit slow but the algorithm is very stable, and it is applicable to a variety of censoring (or truncation) schemes.

Barton [5] generalizes the EM algorithm for the two-sample testing problem, with the cost of further slow down.

Barton considered the following problem: suppose we are given two independent, right censored samples (T_i, δ_i) and (S_j, d_j) where T_i and S_j denote the lifetimes from each sample and δ_i and d_j are the censoring indicators. We want to test the hypothesis

$$H_0 : \int \int g(t, s) dF_T(t) dF_S(s) = \mu .$$

One example of the $g(t, s)$ function is the indicator function $I[t > s]$. The empirical likelihood of the two samples is just the product of their individual sample empirical likelihoods due to the independence assumption. So the NPMLE from the empirical likelihood without constraint is just the two Kaplan–Meier estimators.

Barton used the constrained EM algorithm similar to the above to compute the constrained NPMLE, and finally to form the likelihood ratio. For further details and examples please see Barton [5].

6.4.2 A Recursive Algorithm

Finally, we describe a recursive algorithm here that is better than the above two computational methods: it does not require a lot of memory compared to the sequential quadratic programming method, yet it converges much faster than the EM algorithm. The recursive method is very fast and easily finds the constrained NPMLE, provided the constraint is described in terms of the Lagrange multiplier λ (or tilting parameter). If the constraint is given in terms of μ, then we need to find λ for the required μ. Remember the relation of λ and μ is monotone within the feasible region, so this is not too hard to do.

We recommend this recursive computational method over the other two for computing the constrained Kaplan–Meier estimator and performing the empirical likelihood ratio test. The drawback of this recursive method is that it only works for right censored data, while both the EM algorithm and the sequential quadratic programming methods easily handle right and left censoring, and even interval censoring.

The R function that implements this recursive algorithm is called kmc in a separate package kmc.

We now describe this recursive method of computing the constrained Kaplan–Meier estimator. Recall that the log empirical likelihood for right censored data is (1.24)

$$\log EL_1 = \sum_i \delta_i \log dF(t_i) + (1 - \delta_i) \log[1 - F(t_i)] . \qquad (6.10)$$

Assuming a discrete distribution, with jumps w_i only at the observed times T_i, this becomes

$$\log EL_1 = \sum_{i=1}^{n} \left\{ \delta_i \log w_i + (1 - \delta_i) \log \sum_{j=1}^{n} w_j I[T_j > T_i] \right\} . \qquad (6.11)$$

We notice that without loss of generality, we can assume the smallest T_i is an uncensored one, i.e., the corresponding $\delta = 1$. The reason should be clear from the following: (1) as discussed earlier in Chapter 3, in the EL analysis we may restrict ourselves to those distributions that put probabilities only at the observed, uncensored data points. In other words, we consider only distributions that have the same support as the Kaplan–Meier estimator. It is well-known that Kaplan–Meier puts zero probability on the censored observations; (2) suppose now the smallest observation $T_{(1)}$ is right censored. Then for those discrete distributions (that have the same support as the Kaplan–Meier), the log empirical likelihood function including or excluding the first censored observation is exactly the same; finally, (3) the constraint does not change either including or excluding the first censored observation.

To summarize, if the smallest observed T_i is a right censored one, we may simply delete it and work with the rest of the sample. The empirical likelihood function will be the same and the constraint value will be the same.

Suppose in the observed sample of n survival records (T_i, δ_i) there are k right censored observations. Introduce k new variables, one for each censored T observation, i.e., assume $\delta_j = 0$ and let

$$S_j = \sum_{T_i > T_j} w_i = 1 - \sum_{T_i \leq T_j} w_i . \tag{6.12}$$

This adds k new constraints to the optimization problem of the log empirical likelihood function:

$$S_{j1} = \sum_{i:T_i > T_{j1}} w_i$$

$$\cdots \quad \cdots$$

$$S_{jk} = \sum_{i:T_i > T_{jk}} w_i .$$

With a bit of notational abuse, we write the vector of the k constraints as

$$\mathbf{S} - \sum_{m:T_m >\cdot} w_m = 0.$$

With these k new variables S_j, the log empirical likelihood in terms of the CDF above can be written simply as

$$\log EL(w_i, S_i) = \sum_{\delta_i = 1} \log w_i + \sum_{\delta_i = 0} \log S_i . \tag{6.13}$$

The constraint on the mean is unchanged.

$$\sum_{i=1}^{n} \delta_i g_r(t_i) w_i = \mu_r, \quad r = 1, 2, \cdots, p.$$

The Lagrangian function for the constrained maximum is (without loss of generality assume all $\mu_r = 0$)

$$G = \log EL(w_i, S_i) + \lambda^\top \left(\sum_{\delta_i = 1} g(T_i) w_i \right) - \eta \left(\sum_{i=1}^{n} w_i - 1 \right) - \gamma^\top \left(\mathbf{S} - \sum_{T_i >\cdot} w_i \right) .$$

There are p constraints on the means, so the length of λ is p; one constraint on the summation of w_i equals one, so η is a scalar; and there are k constraints on the newly introduced S_j, so the length of γ is k.

Next we shall take the partial derivatives (with respect to w_i and S_j) and set them to zero. We shall show that $\eta = n$.

Lemma 43 *To maximize the Lagrangian G above, we must have $\eta = n$.*

PROOF: First we compute

$$\frac{\partial G}{\partial S_j} = \frac{1 - \delta_j}{S_j} - \gamma_j \ .$$

Setting the derivative to zero, we have

$$\gamma_j = (1 - \delta_j)/S_j \ . \tag{6.14}$$

Furthermore,

$$\frac{\partial G}{\partial w_k} = \frac{\delta_k}{w_k} + \delta_k \lambda^\top g(T_k) - \eta + \gamma^\top \left(I[T_j < T_k, \delta_j = 0] \right) ,$$

where $I[T_j < T_k, \delta_j = 0]$ is understood as a vector, with T_k fixed, but T_j running through all censored observations.

Setting the derivative to zero, we have (write index k as i)

$$\eta = \frac{\delta_i}{w_i} + \delta_i \lambda^\top g(T_i) + \gamma^\top \left(I[T_j < T_i, \delta_j = 0] \right) \ .$$

Multiply by w_i on both sides and sum:

$$\sum_i w_i \eta = \sum_i \delta_i + \lambda \sum_i \delta_i w_i g(T_i) + \left(\sum_i w_i \gamma^\top I[T_j < T_i, \delta_j = 0] \right) \ .$$

Making use of the other constraints, this simplifies to

$$\eta = (n - k) + 0 + \sum_i w_i \gamma^\top I[T_j < T_i, \delta_j = 0] \ . \tag{6.15}$$

We now focus on the last term above. Plug in the γ_j expression we obtained in (6.14), switch the order of summation, and it is not hard to see that

$$\sum_i w_i \gamma^\top I[T_j < T_i, \delta_j = 0] = \sum_i w_i \left(\sum_j \gamma_j I[T_j < T_i, \delta_j = 0] \right) \tag{6.16}$$

$$= \sum_j \sum_i \frac{w_i I[T_j < T_i, \delta_j = 0]}{S_j} = \sum_j 1 I[\delta_j = 0] = k \ . \tag{6.17}$$

Therefore, Equation (6.15) becomes $\eta = (n - k) + 0 + k$, hence $\eta = n$. $\square$

Using the lemma, $0 = \partial G/\partial w_i$ finally gives rise to

$$w_i = w_i(\lambda) = \frac{\delta_i}{n - \delta_i \lambda^\top g(T_i) - \sum_{j:\delta_j=0} \frac{I[T_j < T_i]}{S_j}} \tag{6.18}$$

which, together with (6.12), provides a recursive computation method for the probabilities w_i (and also S_j) provided λ is given:

1. Starting with the left-most observation, without loss of generality (as noted above) we can assume it is an uncensored point: $\delta_1 = 1$. Thus (6.18) gives

$$w_1 = \frac{1}{n - \lambda^\top g(T_1)} .$$

2. Once we have w_i for all $i \leq m$, we also have all S_j where $T_j < T_{m+1}$ and $\delta_j = 0$, by using $(S_j = 1 - \sum_i I[T_i \leq T_j] w_i)$; then we can compute

$$w_{m+1} = \frac{\delta_{m+1}}{n - \lambda^\top g(T_{m+1}) - \sum_{j: \, \delta_j = 0} \frac{I[T_j < T_{m+1}]}{S_j}} .$$

Therefore, this recursive calculation will give us all w_i and S_j as a function of λ.
Remark: If $\lambda = 0$, then the recursive equation becomes

$$w_{m+1} = \frac{\delta_{m+1}}{n - \sum_{j: \, \delta_j = 0} \frac{I[T_j < T_{m+1}]}{S_j}} \tag{6.19}$$

and $S_j = 1 - \sum_i I[T_i \leq T_j] w_i$. It can be shown that the (jumps of) the Kaplan–Meier estimator satisfy these iteration equations. The key relationship is (5.10). We leave the details to the reader.

Remark: This functional relation of λ to w_i actually is a recursive way of specifying the jumps in the form of (3.7) and (3.15). In Chapter 3 it is asymptotic and not recursive; here it is exact but recursive.

Once we have obtained all the w_i and S_j for a specific λ, the log empirical likelihood is then given by (6.13) with these w_i and S_j. The constrained NPMLE or tilted Kaplan–Meier estimator is just

$$\hat{F}(t) = \sum_{i=1}^n w_i(\lambda) I[T_i \leq t] .$$

We point out that the above calculation is for a given λ. The λ represents the amount of tilting from the Kaplan–Meier. Often we want the constrained Kaplan–Meier estimator with the constraint specified in terms of the mean μ: $\sum_{i=1}^n w_i g(t_i) = \mu$. Therefore, we need to solve the equation(s)

$$\sum_{i=1}^n w_i(\lambda) g(t_i) = \mu$$

to find the exact amount of tilting. The method of solution of this equation is exactly similar to the methods we used to solve the equation for the tilted hazard function in the previous section: bisection for one-dimensional μ, or damped Newton type iterations for multi-dimensional μ. We point out that μ is monotonically related to λ within the feasible region.

The feasible requirement for λ is that $w_i(\lambda) \in [0, 1)$. This translates to the feasible region for μ, in exactly the same fashion for the hazard case. We point out that this is a set of p equations with p unknowns, no matter how big the sample size n is. Compare this to the sequential quadratic programming and EM algorithm, the latter two are used to solve problems with $O(n)$ unknowns where the unknowns are w_i.

Zhou and Yang [143] have conducted some simulation experiments to see how much speedup this new method can achieve when compared to the EM algorithm. In several examples, especially with larger sample sizes and multiple constraints, this recursive method can be several dozen times faster.

This function can be modified to handle a two-sample setup, where the null hypothesis is specified in terms of the difference of the two means from the two samples:

$$H_0 : \int g_1(t)dF_1(t) - \int g_2(t)dF_2(t) = \mu_d .$$

But this can also be handled as follows: introduce an intermediate value a and $b = a - \mu_d$, then turn this into a complete separate two-sample means problem: $H_0 : \int g_1(t)dF_1(t) = a$ and $H_0 : \int g_2(t)dF_2(t) = b$. This can be easily computed by existing R functions (including the recursive algorithm just discussed). A final minimization of the sum of the two empirical likelihood ratios over a would accomplish the original computation problem above.

6.5   EL Testing within the Cox Models and Yang and Prentice Models

As mentioned in Chapter 4, the partial likelihood ratio test for the Cox model, available in all standard software, is the same as the empirical likelihood ratio test when it comes to the hypotheses involving only the regression parameters β. Therefore, the package `emplik` does not include a function for calculating empirical likelihood in this situation.

However, for tests that jointly concern the regression parameter β and the baseline hazard, or just the baseline hazard, we need new software. A function `CoxEL( )` is provided in the package ELYP for computing the log empirical likelihood when we have constraints on the regression parameters as well as on the baseline hazard. The constraint on the baseline is imposed via the equation $\theta = \int g(t)d\Lambda_0(t)$ for the user defined $g(t)$ function. The `CoxEL( )` also computes the constrained baseline hazard. Examples have already appeared in Chapter 4, using this function.

6.5.1   Yang and Prentice Model

For the extension of the Cox model we discussed, i.e., the Yang and Prentice [129] model, all the calculations involved need new software. For some of these calculations we provide a package ELYP. We illustrated the computation using the ggas data in Chapter 4, Section 4.5.

6.6   Testing for AFT Models

6.6.1   The AFT Correlation Model

We discussed this model in Chapter 5. The appropriate empirical likelihood to work with in this model was called "case-wise" empirical likelihood. First, the computation of the estimator or the solution to the estimating equation (5.7) is provided by R function WRegEst( ). The weights used are the jumps of the Kaplan–Meier specified in (5.9).

The calculation of the log empirical likelihood ratio for testing the regression parameter β is done by calling the R function WRegTest( ), which will set up the estimating functions in (5.17) and call el.cen.EM2( ) to test the hypothesis about β.

6.6.2   The AFT Regression Model

We discuss the computation only of the Buckley–James estimation method. The Buckley–James estimator or solution to the estimating equations (5.3) can be computed by R function bj( ) from the R package rms. However, the variance estimator provided by this function is not correct. Nevertheless, the function can provide a ballpark estimate (search area) when we are inverting the EL test to get the EL based confidence region. This function always requires an intercept term in the regression model.

We provide a function BJnoint( ) in the emplik package. It does similar calculations to bj( ) of the rms package, except it does not provide a variance estimator, and checking of iteration convergence is entirely left to the user. The Buckley–James iteration computation may not converge no matter how many iterations are done. The estimators may oscillate between two values or loop through several values. See Currie [17].

Although the name BJnoint( ) indicates that it does not include an intercept term in the regression model by default, you may, of course, include a column of 1s in your design matrix to force an intercept term. In this case, the estimator should agree with bj( ), provided the iteration converges.

Calculation of the empirical likelihood ratio for testing β is done by the function el.cen.EM2( ). However, we need to calculate the Buckley–James estimating equations of the second form in (5.3). For this, the emplik package provides a function bj.test( ). It will calculate the estimating function in the form (5.3) and then call el.cen.EM2( ) to test it.

Example 25 *We saw in Chapter 5 the example of computing the Buckley–James estimator for the AFT regression model with Stanford heart transplant data. We also showed a plot of the joint confidence region of the intercept and slope, (β_1, β_2). The estimator of (β_1, β_2) is $(3.5275, -0.0199)$.*

Here we show how to find the confidence interval of a one-dimensional parameter defined by $h(\beta_1, \beta_2)$. This function does not have to be a linear function but the calculation in this example uses a linear function of β_1 and β_2. For example, the

mean value for a 50-year-old patient is, from the AFT regression model, $\beta_1 + 50\beta_2$.
So, we take $h(\beta_1, \beta_2) = \beta_1 + 50\beta_2$.

In the following stanford5 *is the Stanford heart transplant data we formed in*
Example 21.

```
library(ELYP)
Bfun <- function(b1, b2){b1+50*b2}
BJLLR <- function(para, dataMat) {
      bjtest(y=log10(dataMat[,2]), d=dataMat[,3],
                x=cbind(1,dataMat[,4]), beta=para)
}


BJfindL2(NPmle=c(3.5275, -0.0199), ConfInt=c(1, 0.04),
              LLRfn=BJLLR, Betafun=Bfun, dataMat=stanford5)
## ...
## $Lower
## [1] 2.395945
## ...


BJfindU2(NPmle=c(3.5275, -0.0199), ConfInt=c(1, 0.04),
              LLRfn=BJLLR, Betafun=Bfun, dataMat=stanford5)
## ...
## $Upper
## [1] 2.669052
## ...
```

We see that the 95% confidence interval for $\beta_1 + 50\beta_2$ is $(2.395945, 2.669052)$.

The input NPmle *is the Buckley–James estimator we obtained in Chapter 5 for β_1*
and β_2. Here they do not have to be exact. They just provide a starting point for the
search. The input ConfInt *is used as the initial step size of the search. Ideal values*
should be (approximately) the half length of the confidence interval for β_1 and β_2.
We can estimate these by looking at the contour plot of the joint confidence region
for β_1, β_2. Again, they do not have to be exact.

6.7 Empirical Likelihood for Overdetermined Estimating Equations

For censored data there is no ready R-code to compute the empirical likelihood with
overdetermined estimating equations. However, in the case of k parameters and $k+1$
estimating equations, the required calculation is just a minimization of likelihoods
over a single parameter. This is often quite easy. Our example in Chapter 2 is based
on this case.

For uncensored data, we might be able to use the function from R package gmm,
which is geared mostly toward econometrics. In addition to the generalized method
of moments, it also includes the empirical likelihood calculations for the overdetermined estimating equation setting.

6.8   Testing Part of the Parameter Vector

In a multiple regression model, suppose the parameters are $\beta = (\beta_1, \beta_2)$ and suppose also we already have an empirical likelihood ratio for testing the whole vector β:

$$H_0 : \beta = \beta_0 .$$

Now we would like to test part of the parameter vector: let $\beta = (\beta_1, \beta_2)$ and consider

$$H_{01} : \beta_1 = \beta_{10} .$$

This hypothesis can be tested by the profile likelihood method: we profile out the nuisance parameter β_2. Therefore, the profile likelihood is

$$W(\beta_1) = \inf_{\beta_2} W(\beta_1, \beta_2) ,$$

where $W(\beta_1, \beta_2)$ is the -2 log likelihood ratio for testing the parameter (β_1, β_2) and $W(\beta_1)$ is the -2 log likelihood ratio for testing β_1 alone. This problem is not specific to the empirical likelihood but common to all likelihood ratio tests.

For a parameter that is defined by $h(\beta_1, \beta_2)$, we can similarly use the profile technique. Due to the invariance of likelihoods with respect to the parameter transformation, we may view the likelihood in terms of the new parameters $h(\beta_1, \beta_2)$ and $g(\beta_1, \beta_2)$. We then need to "profile out" the second parameter $g(\beta_1, \beta_2)$ to get the -2 log likelihood ratio for $h(\beta_1, \beta_2)$ alone.

We remind the reader that this profile process is easy to describe but its implementation can be challenging. Especially in the multi-dimensional case (e.g., profile out a six-dimensional parameter vector) the calculation can be slow.

Another related problem is to invert the likelihood ratio test to obtain confidence intervals for each parameter alone (instead of a joint confidence region). This involves profiling the -2 log likelihood ratio down to one parameter and then inverting the test to obtain the confidence interval.

We have already seen examples of profiling the empirical likelihood ratio and using the function findU2 to invert the test, etc.

6.9   Intermediate Parameters

Sometimes it is easier to compute the empirical likelihood if we introduce some additional intermediate parameters. After we obtain the log empirical likelihood ratio, we may then profile out the intermediate parameter. We saw some examples of this in previous chapters, when we tested the ratio of two survival probabilities. Let us look at one more example.

Example 26 *Given a sample of n i.i.d. observations $X_1, \cdots, X_n$, we wish to use the empirical likelihood ratio to test the hypothesis*

$$H_0 : Var(X) = V^0 .$$

The null hypothesis in the discrete case becomes a constraint equation

$$V^0 = \sum_{i=1}^{n} p_i \left(x_i - \sum_j p_j x_j \right)^2$$

for the empirical likelihood $EL = \prod p_i$.

Maximization of the empirical likelihood with the constraint cannot be performed directly by el.test( )*, because the variance definition also involves the nuisance parameter of mean, and the constraint equation is not linear in p_i.*

However, if we introduce an intermediate parameter

$$\sum p_i x_i = \mu \,,$$

then the hypothesis

$$H_{00} : Var(X) = V^0, \quad E(X) = \mu$$

can be handled by the el.test( )*. The resulting log likelihood ratio will have a chi square with two degrees of freedom under the null hypothesis H_{00}. But of course we do not know the true value of μ.*

Denote the -2 log likelihood ratio for testing the H_{00} above as $W(\mu)$. We shall profile out the intermediate parameter μ by minimizing $W(\mu)$ over μ. After the profiling, the log empirical likelihood ratio will have asymptotically a chi square distribution with one degree of freedom under the null hypothesis H_0.

In the following we test the hypothesis that the waiting time of the Old Faithful Geyser has variance equal to 180. Technically, we could also work with right censored data, but variance is rarely used to describe censored survival distributions.

```
data(faithful)
xvec <- faithful$waiting
mean(xvec)
## [1] 70.89706
var(xvec)
## [1] 184.8233
ELH00 <- function(x, m, V0) {
        xmat <- cbind(x, (x-m)^2)
        el.test(x=xmat, mu=c(m, V0))
}
ELH00(x=xvec, m=70, V0=180)
optim(70, fn=function(m, x, V0)
            {ELH00(x, m=m, V0)$"-2LLR"}, x=xvec, V0=180)
## $par
## [1] 71.04932
##
## $value
## [1] 0.1618861
##
```

So the -2 log empirical likelihood ratio for testing $H_0 : Var(X) = 180$ is 0.1618861. *This corresponds to a p-value of* 0.6874259, *since* $P(\chi_1^2 > 0.1618861) =$ 0.6874259.

The topics in the following section can also be viewed as applications of the intermediate parameter method.

6.10   Lorenz Curve and Trimmed Mean

Without loss of generality, assume the random variables of interest in this section are always nonnegative.

For right censored survival data, the parameter of *mean survival* is seldom used. One reason is that the mean is very much dependent on the tail behavior of the survival curve, and the Kaplan–Meier survival curve has large variability in the right tail, making the mean estimator unstable.

A possible remedy is to use the truncated mean or trimmed mean. We discuss trimmed mean here. Usually the *trimmed mean* refers to a mean symmetrically trimmed from both upper and lower tails. But for survival data or data with a skewed distribution, trimming only the right tail also makes sense.

For example, in economics, income distribution resides on the nonnegative half line and is right skewed with a long right tail. A mean trimmed only on the right tail makes a lot of sense here. In fact, there are many measures of income inequality based on right tail trimmed means.

In economics the generalized Lorenz curve is defined as follows. For an (income) CDF, $F(\cdot)$, that resides on the nonnegative half line, define the function

$$GLC(p) = \int_0^{\xi(p)} x dF(x) , \quad \text{for } 0 \le p \le 1$$

where $\xi(p)$ is the quantile $F(\xi(p)) = p$. So, the generalized Lorenz curve at a given p is just the upper tail trimmed mean.

On the other hand, the Lorenz curve itself is defined as

$$LC(p) = \frac{GLC(p)}{\mu} ,$$

where μ is the mean of $F(\cdot)$. The area between the 45 degree diagonal line and the Lorenz curve summarizes how much the Lorenz curve sags below the 45 degree line (a measure of income inequality). Twice the area is called the Gini index, another measure of income inequality.

Nonparametric estimation of the GLC, LC and the Gini index has been discussed by many authors. Gastwirth [32] has defined and studied the nonparametric estimation of the (generalized) Lorenz curve and Gini index.

Beach and Davidson [7] showed the joint normality of the estimators of Lorenz curve ordinates. Chakraborti [11] constructed joint confidence intervals for the Lorenz curve ordinates.

Statistical inference for the Lorenz curve for censored data was studied by Cowell and Victoria-Feser [14]. Gigliaranno and Muliere [34] used the Bayes nonparametric method to estimate the Lorenz curve from censored data.

We discuss first the empirical likelihood ratio test and construction of a confidence interval of $GLC(p)$ for a given $p \in (0,1)$, based on a right censored sample from an independent censoring model with survival distribution $F(\cdot)$.

Qin et al. [91] also proposed using empirical likelihood to test the $GLC(p)$. But our approach here is different, and has some unique features: (1) We allow randomly right censored data, which is useful since the income data are often subject to right censoring due to confidentiality issues. (2) The limiting distribution of our empirical likelihood ratio under the null hypothesis is a regular chi square. In addition to the simplicity of setting up the critical values for the test, this also suggests some kind of optimality compared to the scaled chi squared distribution obtained in Qin et al. [91]. In fact, the empirical likelihood proposed by Qin et al. is a "plug-in" likelihood, as we discuss in Chapter 7. Please see Chapter 7 for the optimality discussion. (3) It is easy to generalize our method to get confidence regions for multiple parameters (i.e., multiple Lorenz curve ordinates or other quantities). Here we shall describe briefly how to test simultaneously the Lorenz curve ordinates at two places p_1 and p_2. The resulting empirical likelihood ratio will have a chi square distribution with two degrees of freedom under the null hypothesis.

We now focus on testing, for a given $p \in (0,1)$, the hypothesis

$$H_0 : GLC(p) = \theta \qquad (6.20)$$

given a random sample of right censored observations.

We compute the test statistic in two steps. First we test the hypothesis, for some given τ,

$$H_{00} : F(\tau) = p \quad \text{and} \quad \int_0^\tau x dF(x) = \theta . \qquad (6.21)$$

This hypothesis can also be written as

$$H_{00} : F^{-1}(p) = \tau \quad \text{and} \quad \int_0^{F^{-1}(p)} x dF(x) = \theta .$$

The empirical likelihood ratio for testing this hypothesis can be computed using el.cen.EM2( ). Assuming τ is the "true" value, the limiting null distribution of the resulting log empirical likelihood ratio has a chi square distribution with two degrees of freedom, since there are two constraints. The true value of τ is the population pth quantile of F. We of course do not know the true τ. We used this method of introducing an intermediate parameter τ in Section 3.5 for equality of k medians.

Next we view the resulting empirical likelihood ratio as a function of τ and profile out τ (minimizing over τ). The minimum value obtained is the (profile) empirical likelihood ratio $W = \inf_\tau W(\tau)$, suitable for testing

$$H_0 : GLC(p) = \theta ,$$

where W has asymptotically a chi square distribution with one degree of freedom under the null hypothesis (6.20).

In the R example below, we use a Pareto distribution with shape parameter $\alpha = 2$ to generate randomly simulated income data.

```r
library(emplik)
sizeN <- 5000
set.seed(123)
x <- 1/sqrt(runif(sizeN))
cen <-  1.5 + 5* runif(sizeN)
x <- pmin(x, cen)
d <- as.numeric(x <= cen)

trimP <- 0.8  # We fix p at 0.8.
thetaP <- 2*(1 - sqrt(1-0.8))
tau0 <- 2.2
LLR1 <- function(tau, trimP, thetaP, x, d) {
    gfun1 <- function(x, tau){ as.numeric(x <= tau) }
    gfun2 <- function(x, tau){ x[x >= tau] <- 0; x }
    gfun12 <- function(x, tau){
                    cbind(gfun1(x, tau), gfun2(x, tau))}
    el.cen.EM2(x=x, d=d,  fun=gfun12,
                    mu=c(trimP, thetaP), tau=tau)$"-2LLR"
}
LLR1(tau=tau0, trimP, thetaP, x, d)
```

In the above example we are attempting to test the hypothesis $H_0 : GLC(0.8) = 2*(1 - \sqrt{1-0.8})$. We get the likelihood ratio for a fixed τ above. Next we need to minimize over all possible τ. We first note that the log empirical likelihood ratio is a piecewise constant function of τ. Thus we may just search τ over strategically placed values, checking one τ between any two consecutive observations. Hence we need only search a maximum of $(n-1)$ values to find the minimum (often fewer). The "true" value of τ in this case for the Pareto distribution is 2.23. In reality we do not know the true value. But after some trial runs, it is easy to set an interval to search the minimum with respect to τ, due to the convexity property. In our example, we shall search over the τ values within (2, 2.4). As Fig. 6.1 shows, the minimum is well within this interval.

```r
xsort <- sort(x)
xsort2 <- xsort[(xsort > 2) & (xsort < 2.4)]
tauvec <- (xsort2[-1] + xsort2[-length(xsort2)])/2
llrvec <- rep(NA, length(tauvec))

for(i in 1:length(tauvec))
    llrvec[i] <- LLR1(tauvec[i], trimP, thetaP, x, d)

min(llrvec)
##  [1] 2.602961
```

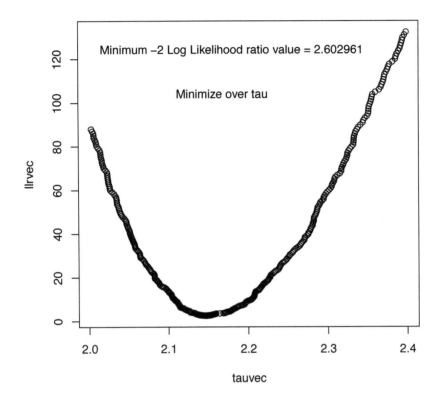

Figure 6.1: Profile for minimizing over τ. Minimum happens near $\tau = 2.14$.

```
which.min(llrvec)
## [1] 172
llrvec[ which.min(llrvec) ]
## [1] 2.602961
```

The *p*-value of this (profile) -2 log likelihood ratio value can be computed using the chi square distribution with one degree of freedom.

```
1-pchisq(2.602961, df=1)
## [1] 0.1066643
```

Let us now study inference of the Lorenz curve. Notice that the hypothesis, for given *p*,

$$H_0: LC(p) = \phi$$

is equivalent to

$$H_0 : \ GLC(p) = \phi\mu$$

and again is equivalent to

$$GLC(p) - \phi\mu = 0 \ .$$

This last form of the hypothesis can be tested by using el.cen.EM2( ), in two steps similar to the test of GLC above.

First, we test, for a given τ, the hypothesis

$$H_{00} : \ F(\tau) = p \quad \text{and} \quad \int_0^\tau x dF(x) - \phi\mu = 0 \ .$$

Let us define two functions

$$g_1(x, \tau) = I[x \le \tau], \quad g_2(x, \tau) = xI[x \le \tau] - \phi x$$

then the above H_{00} is just

$$H_{00} : \ \int_0^\infty g_1(x, \tau) dF(x) = p, \quad \text{and} \quad \int_0^\infty g_2(x, \tau) dF(x) = 0 \ .$$

This is precisely the form of hypothesis that the function el.cen.EM2( ) is designed to handle. Denote the resulting empirical likelihood ratio for testing H_{00} as $W(\tau)$, then $W = \inf_\tau W(\tau)$ will be the (profile) empirical likelihood ratio for testing the hypothesis

$$H_0 : \ LC(p) = \phi \ .$$

Also, under the null hypothesis W has an asymptotic distribution of chi square with one degree of freedom. A confidence interval can be obtained by inverting the test.

Testing the Lorenz curve ordinates at several different locations can be done similarly. We briefly describe the procedure here. Suppose $0 < p_1 < p_2 < 1$ are two given points. For given $\phi_1 < \phi_2$, we shall test the hypothesis

$$H_0 : \ LC(p_1) = \phi_1 \quad \text{and} \quad LC(p_2) = \phi_2, \tag{6.22}$$

using the empirical likelihood ratio as follows. First we introduce two intermediate values τ_1 and τ_2, and for the two given points $0 < \tau_1 < \tau_2 < \infty$, we use el.cen.EM2( ) to test the hypothesis

$$H_{00} : \quad F(\tau_1) = p_1; \ \int_0^\infty (xI[x \le \tau_1] - \phi_1 x) dF(x) = 0; \tag{6.23}$$

$$F(\tau_2) = p_2; \ \int_0^\infty (xI[x \le \tau_2] - \phi_2 x) dF(x) = 0 \ .$$

The resulting log empirical likelihood ratio has an asymptotic chi square df = 4 distribution under the null hypothesis H_{00}, provided τ_1 and τ_2 are the "true" values. We denote the likelihood ratio statistic as $W(\tau_1, \tau_2)$. The final step is to minimize (profile) the W over all possible $0 < \tau_1 < \tau_2 < \infty$. The resulting $W =$

$\inf_{\tau_1 < \tau_2} W(\tau_1, \tau_2)$ will have a chi square distribution with two degrees of freedom under the null hypothesis H_0, asymptotically. And the profile W is suitable for testing the hypothesis (6.22).

TRIMMED MEAN

The $GLC(p)$ is essentially a one-sided trimmed mean. In other applications, two-sided, symmetrically trimmed means are more common. It is a compromise between a mean and a median.

Given a CDF $F(t)$, the p-trimmed mean $(0 \leq p < 0.5)$ is defined as

$$\mu(p) = \frac{1}{1 - 2p} \int_{\xi(p)}^{\eta(p)} t\, dF(t), \quad \text{where } F(\xi(p)) = p; \; F(\eta(p)) = 1 - p \,.$$

Given an i.i.d. sample of size n from F, an estimator of the trimmed mean based on the sample is

$$\hat{\mu}(p) = \frac{1}{1 - 2p} \int_a^b t\, d\hat{F}_n(t), \quad \text{where } \hat{F}_n(a) = p; \; \hat{F}_n(b) = 1 - p \,, \tag{6.24}$$

where $\hat{F}_n(t)$ is the empirical distribution function. Due to discreteness of $\hat{F}_n$, we usually restrict p to be one of the values in the list $\{1/n, 2/n, \cdots\}$.

When available data are right censored, the above estimate, (6.24), of the trimmed mean is still valid except $\hat{F}_n(t)$ there should be replaced by the Kaplan–Meier estimator constructed from the right censored data. The following testing procedure will also be the same except the el.test( ) function should be replaced by el.cen.EM2( ). For presentation simplicity, we use the uncensored case in the following description.

For a given $0 < p < 0.5$, we would like to test the hypothesis

$$H_0 : \mu(p) = \mu^0 \tag{6.25}$$

using the empirical likelihood ratio.

We proceed as follows: introduce two intermediate parameters, r and s with $r < s$ and consider the hypothesis

$$H_{00} : F(r) = p, \; F(s) = 1 - p, \; \frac{1}{1 - 2p} \int_r^s t\, dF(t) = \mu^0 \,.$$

The empirical likelihood ratio for testing this (three equalities) hypothesis can be obtained using the procedure described in Chapter 1 or Chapter 3 if the data are right censored. The resulting log empirical likelihood ratio, $W(r, s)$, will have an asymptotic null (H_{00}) distribution of chi square with three degrees of freedom.

Finally, we shall profile out the intermediate parameters r and s by minimizing $W(r, s)$ over all pairs $r < s$.

In the profiled log empirical likelihood ratio, $\min_{r < s} W(r, s)$ is suitable for testing the hypothesis (6.25) and has a chi square one degree of freedom distribution under (6.25) asymptotically.

We also note that, due to discreteness, in the search of a minimum we need only work with r and s points that are placed between actual observed sample values of X_i. Often we can search a much smaller list than this due to the convexity of the log likelihood function. This speeds up the search.

Example 27 *For simplicity we take a dataset without censoring. If the data are right censored, we just need to replace the empirical distribution $\hat{F}_n(t)$ in the above discussion by the Kaplan–Meier estimator, and use* el.cen.EM2( ) *instead of* el.test( ) *in computing the log empirical likelihood ratio below.*

In the following example we use the trim $p = 0.05 = 3/60$ and test $\mu^0 = 50$.

```
data(nhtemp)
xvec <- sort(nhtemp)
trimP <- 3/length(xvec)
mu0 <- 50
HOOEL <- function(x, r, s, p, mu) {
    xmat <- cbind(as.numeric(x <= r),
                  as.numeric(x <= s),
                  (x*as.numeric((r < x)&(x <= s)))/(1-2*p) )
    el.test(xmat, mu=c(p, 1-p, mu) )
}
HOOEL(x=xvec, r=49, s=53.02, p=trimP, mu=mu0)
## $'-2LLR'
## [1] 73.53101
## ...
N <- length(xvec)
INDX <- (xvec[-N] + xvec[-1])/2
temp <- matrix(NA, nrow=(N-2), ncol=(N-2))
for(i in 1:(N-2))
    for(j in (i+1):(N-1))
        temp[i,(j-1)] <- HOOEL(x=xvec, r=INDX[i],
                        s=INDX[j], p=trimP, mu=mu0)$"-2LLR"
min(temp, na.rm=TRUE)
## [1] 38.57715
```

This result corresponds to a small p-value of $P(\chi_1^2 > 38.57715) = 5.263151e - 10$. Preliminary calculation should probably be used to narrow down the search area and speed up the calculation. Confidence intervals for the trimmed mean can be constructed by inverting the test.

So far we have not payed attention to smoothing. As Chen and Hall [12] showed, in the uncensored data case smoothing can improve the accuracy of the chi square approximation in the quantile empirical likelihood. Here in the trimming part, we do deal with the quantiles of the unknown CDF as the trimming proportions. Therefore, smoothing is expected to play a similar role as in Chen and Hall [12]. Extensive simulations are currently under way. Different smoothing window and type of smoothing kernel shall be compared.

Our approach of EL analysis for the trimmed mean has the advantage of yielding a regular chi square distribution under the null hypothesis; thus it is easy to use and the generalization to the censored data case is straightforward. There is no asymptotic variance to estimate. Plus, the asymptotic null distribution of a regular chi square suggests that the confidence region obtained by inverting the EL test has certain optimality property. See Chapter 7 for more discussion.

A different empirical likelihood analysis for trimmed mean was considered by Qin and Tsao [90] and Velina and Valeinis [121]. However, the log empirical likelihood ratio of their approach has a scaled chi square distribution asymptotically under the null hypothesis. Their approach can be viewed as a "plug-in" empirical likelihood, discussed in detail in Chapter 7.

6.11 Confidence Intervals

The previous sections discussed calculations of empirical likelihood ratio tests for various situations. In practice, we often also want to calculate a confidence region or confidence interval. It is conceptually simple to invert a likelihood ratio test to obtain a confidence interval or confidence region. If the likelihood ratio test statistic for the hypothesis $H_0 : \theta = a$ is denoted as $-2 \log ELR(a)$, that is, H_0 is rejected if $-2 \log ELR(a) > C$, then

$$\{a| \ -2 \log ELR(a) \leq C\}$$

is the confidence region for θ. In other words, the acceptance region of the test is the confidence region. The constant C is often chosen as the 95th percentile of the chi square distribution with p degrees of freedom, where $p = dim(\theta)$, due to the Wilks theorem. For smaller samples, the chi square distribution may be replaced by other better approximations like F-distribution with n and one degree of freedom. In this case the nominal coverage probability of the resulting confidence region is 95%.

But in reality this inversion can be tedious and computationally intensive. For example, how would you specify a four-dimensional confidence region? The difficulty also lies with the property that these confidence regions are NOT simply the ellipsoid (as the Wald confidence regions are), which can be characterized by the location vector and the dispersion matrix. The confidence regions from inverting the empirical likelihood ratio test have no fixed shape. This is an advantage: the data driven shape of the confidence region. But a shape/region in four or higher dimensions is hard to describe.

Finding an effective way to accurately compute the confidence interval/region can be tricky and depends on each individual case. We give several examples below. In these examples, if the confidence region is for a two-dimensional parameter, then we use a plot to show the region. However, for higher dimensions, instead of trying to characterize a high dimensional confidence region, we compute several one-dimensional confidence intervals, i.e., instead of a four-dimensional confidence region, we give four confidence intervals for four individual parameters (or profiling).

Remark: This difficulty is not specific to *empirical likelihood*, but also to regular parametric likelihood analysis. So, some of the examples below are actually for regular likelihood ratio tests.

When the empirical likelihood ratio test is about a single parameter, the related confidence interval is relatively easier to find and we provide a function findUL in the package emplik to help find the confidence interval.

When the empirical likelihood ratio tests are for two parameters (a two-dimensional parameter), θ_1 and θ_2, we can either produce a contour plot showing the confidence region, or we may want a confidence interval for one new parameter, say $f(\theta_1, \theta_2)$. The latter computation is more involved. We give several examples for a simple, general search method. Better methods could be found by taking advantage of the special property of the $f(\theta_1, \theta_2)$ function involved, or knowledge of the range of the parameter θ_1, θ_2.

For tests of more parameters (dimension p larger than 3), a similar idea could be applied theoretically, but the search becomes slower. This is similar to the curse of dimensionality.

Example 28 *(Confidence interval for survival probability at fixed time τ)*
  We use the lung *dataset in the package* survival. *The estimator of the survival probability is given by the Kaplan–Meier estimator. We take $\tau = 365.25$.*

```
library(emplik)
library(survival)
data(lung)
myfunP <- function(theta,x,d){
el.cen.EM2(x=x, d=d, fun=function(t){
                        as.numeric(t>365.25)}, mu=theta)}
findUL(step=0.01,fun=myfunP,MLE=0.4,x=lung$time,
                        d=lung$status-1)
## $Low
## [1] 0.3402327
##
## $Up
## [1] 0.4799405
```

In the output you can find the 95% Wilks confidence interval based on the Kaplan–Meier estimator of the survival probability at $\tau = 365.25$ days is $(0.3402327, 0.4799405)$.

A few comments are in order. (1) For the 90% confidence interval, an optional command of level=2.705543 *can be added to the function* findUL. *Notice here the degree of freedom is one. The default level is 3.84 for a 95% confidence interval. (2) The MLE is set to be 0.4. Actually the true MLE of survival at $\tau = 365.25$ is 0.409. This program does not need the exact MLE of survival at τ. A good enough approximation often works fine. The indication if an approximation works is that in the output,* Lvalue *and* Uvalue *are both approximately equal to the level you set (here the default, so $= 3.84$). (3) The step $= 0.01$ seems to work well if the final confidence intervals are all within $(0, 1)$, as is the case here. It is the search step size.*

You may want to set it to a larger value if your confidence interval (upper/lower) limits are expected to be more than 10 units away from the MLE, say.

Example 29 *(Survival probability from a Weibull model) Using the same dataset as above, we seek to fit a two-parameter Weibull model to the data: λ-scale parameter, β-shape parameter. We want to find the 90% confidence interval for the survival probability if a Weibull distribution with two parameters is used: the parameter of interest is $\theta = \exp(-(\lambda \times t)^\beta)$, where we take $t = 365.25 \times 1.5 = 547.875$.*

1. We first look at values of (λ, β) and see which values are "likely" and which are "unlikely." The criterion is whether the -2 log likelihood ratio for this pair of (λ, β) parameters is less than 2.70 (likely) and which pairs have larger than 2.70 (unlikely). Recall 2.70 is the 90th percentile of the chi square df = 1 distribution. Sometimes we call them "inside" (=likely) vs "outside" = unlikely.

2. For those "likely" values of (λ, β)s, we compute $\exp(-(\lambda \times t)^\beta)$; call them θs.

3. The confidence interval is just $\min(\theta)$ and $\max(\theta)$.

First, define a function to compute the log likelihood for the Weibull model with censored data:

```
weiloglik <- function(lam, beta, x, d){
   sum(d*(log(beta)+beta*log(lam)+(beta-1)*log(x))) -
     sum((lam*x)^beta)
}
```

Next we need to compute the -2 log likelihood ratio. To this end we first need to find the maximum value this Weibull log likelihood can achieve.

From the `survreg( )` *function of the R* `survival` *package, we can compute the MLE: lamMLE $= 0.002393727$, betaMLE $= 1.31684$. Then the maximum value of the Weibull likelihood can be computed as*

```
weiloglik(lam=0.002393727, beta=1.31684, x=time, d=status)
## gives -1153.851
```

Now the likelihood ratio:

```
weiLR <- function(lam, beta, x, d, maxValue= -1153.851) {
      temp <- -2*( weiloglik(lam=lam, beta=beta, x=x, d=d)
                                        - maxValue )
list("-2LLR"=temp )
}
```

The R code to produce the contour plot:

```
xivec <- 1:100/25000        ### set up the region to
yivec <- 1:100/200 +1       ### draw the plot. It
zmat <- matrix(NA, 100, 100)   ### should be near the
for(i in 1:100) for(j in 1:100) ### center (=MLE).
```

```
        zmat[i,j] <- weiLR(lam=xivec[i], beta=yivec[j],
                    x=lung$time,d=lung$status-1)$"-2LLR"
contour(x=xivec, y=yivec, z=zmat, level=c(0.5,1,2,2.7,3.84),
                                xlab="lambda", ylab="beta")
```

Check the contour plot to make sure we have covered the confidence region (i.e., those with zmat *smaller than 2.70, otherwise adjust* xivec *and/or* yivec*).*
Computation of all the θ's:

```
Smat <- matrix(NA, 100, 100)
for(i in 1:100) for(j in 1:100)
        Smat[i,j] <- exp(-(xivec[i]*365.25*1.5)^yivec[j])
```

This computes all the theta values from "likely" and "unlikely" parameters. We finally pick those corresponding to "likely" parameter values and find the maximum and minimum, which is the 90% confidence interval:

```
likelySurv <- Smat[ zmat <= 2.70 ]
min(likelySurv)
max(likelySurv)
```

Example 30 *(Ratio of cumulative hazards from two independent samples) We take the* lung *data from the* survival *package, and separate it into two samples according to the covariate* sex*.*

```
data(lung)
time1 <- lung$time[lung$sex == 1]
time2 <- lung$time[lung$sex == 2]
d1 <- lung$status[lung$sex == 1] - 1
d2 <- lung$status[lung$sex == 2] - 1

mymedfun <- function(t, M){as.numeric(t > M)}
S1vec <- 1:100/400 + 0.22
S2vec <- 1:100/250 + 0.3
zmat <- matrix(NA, 100, 100)
for(i in 1:100)for(j in 1:100)
    zmat[i,j]<-el.cen.EM2(x=time1,d=d1,fun=mymedfun,
                    mu=S1vec[i],M=365.25)$"-2LLR" +
            el.cen.EM2(x=time2,d=d2,fun=mymedfun,
                    mu=S2vec[j],M=365.25)$"-2LLR"
contour(x=S1vec, y=S2vec, z=zmat, level=c(0.3, 2.7, 3.8, 5))

Smat <- zmat
for(i in 1:100)for(j in 1:100)
        Smat[i,j] <- log(S1vec[i])/log(S2vec[j])
```

```
likelyV <- Smat[zmat <= 2.705543]
max(likelyV)
## [1] 2.421312
min(likelyV)
## [1] 1.205018
```

Therefore, the 90% confidence interval for the ratio of cumulative hazards at $\tau = 365.25$ *days is (1.205018, 2.421312).*

Comment: Here we estimate the cumulative hazard by $-\log(\hat{S}(t))$, *where* $\hat{S}(t)$ *is the Kaplan–Meier estimator. If you would rather use the Nelson–Aalen estimator to estimate the cumulative hazard, you should do*

```
myfun2 <- function(t){as.numeric(t <= 365.25)}
H1vec <- -log(S1vec)
H2vec <- -log(S2vec)
for(i in 1:100) for(j in1:100) zmat[i,j] <-
        emplikH1.test(x=time1,d=d1,theta=H1vec[i],
                                fun=myfun2)$"-2LLR" +
        emplikH1.test(x=time2,d=d2,theta=H2vec[j],
                                fun=myfun2)$"-2LLR"

for(i in 1:100)for(j in 1:100)
                Smat[i,j] <- H1vec[i]/H2vec[j]

likelyV <- Smat[zmat <= 2.705543]
max(likelyV)
## [1] 2.451968
min(likelyV)
## [1] 1.196852
```

6.12   Historic Note and Generalizations

The case-wise EL approach (i.e., the estimating equation and the related empirical likelihood ratio) to the AFT correlation model can be easily modified to accommodate M-estimators. One such example is the quantile estimator. Zhou et al. [141] include a quantile regression using a similar approach, while Kim et al. [55] studied quantile regression for the residual life.

For the median AFT correlation model, Huang et al. [45] studied the large sample properties of the case weight estimator. They show the estimator is consistent and asymptotically normally distributed.

Owen's book [81] mentions at least one unpublished paper related to EL analysis for the trimmed mean, by La Rocca. However, I am unable to locate a copy of the paper.

The trimmed mean definition we used may have some ambiguity when there are tied observations. The key is that $\hat{F}^{-1}(p)$ may not be defined satisfactorily when there is a flat interval for $\hat{F}$ with value p. In those cases, smoothing is seen as a solution. We may either smooth the indicator function that defines the $\hat{F}$, as Chen and Hall [12] did, or directly smooth the likelihood function.

6.13   Exercises

Exercise 6.1 *Show that the jumps of the Kaplan–Meier estimator satisfy the recursive equation (6.19). Hint: make use of (5.10).*

Exercise 6.2 *Show that $w(\lambda)$ as given in (6.6) is a monotone function of λ. Find the interval of λ such that the corresponding $p_i(\lambda)$ are all between 0 and 1.*

Exercise 6.3 *In the context of Example 27, obtain a 90% confidence interval for the trimmed mean.*

Chapter 7

Optimality of Empirical Likelihood and Plug-in Empirical Likelihood

In this chapter we discuss the optimality of empirical likelihood tests via their induced confidence regions. The optimality of parametric likelihood ratio tests is well-known. Although not formally stated, it is more or less implied that the optimality of likelihood ratio tests also carries over to empirical likelihood ratio tests. However, there are many variations of the empirical likelihood approach in the literature. If we are not careful, some variations of empirical likelihood tests may not be optimal. The induced confidence regions can be drastically different.

Since the empirical likelihood functions we have discussed so far in this book are identical to the nonparametric likelihoods, the maximum empirical likelihood estimators will be the same as the nonparametric maximum likelihood estimators (NPMLE). The optimality of the NPMLEs is also well-known. Therefore, when study the variations of empirical likelihood, it is obvious that if a type of pseudo empirical likelihood is not maximized at the NPMLE, it cannot be optimal. However, even if a pseudo empirical likelihood is maximized at the genuine NPMLE, it does not imply that it will produce an optimal test or confidence region automatically. The optimality also depends on the curvature or the second derivative of the EL at the maximum location.

7.1 Pseudo Empirical Likelihood Ratio Test

Recall we have right censored data from random independent censorship model $T_i = \min(X_i, C_i)$ and $\delta_i = I[X_i \le C_i]$. A class of pseudo empirical likelihood test for right censored data is often based on the following lemma.

Lemma 44 *For any function $g(\cdot)$ such that $Eg(X_i)$ is well defined, we have $Eg(X_i) = EZ_i$ where*

$$Z_i = \frac{g(T_i)\delta_i}{1 - G_0(T_i)} ,$$

and $G_0(\cdot)$ is the CDF of the censoring variable C_i, provided that $1 - G_0(T_i) > 0$ almost surely (a.s.).

PROOF: *Notice that for computing the expectation, we can condition on* $\delta_i = 1$. *Thus*

$$EZ_i = \int \frac{g(t)}{1 - G_0(t)}[1 - G_0(t)]dF(t) = \int g(t)dF(t) = Eg(X_i) \ .$$

$\square$

This transformation in Lemma 44 sometimes is called the "inverse censoring probability" weighting scheme, since we may view this as a multiplicative weight $\delta_i/[1 - G_0(T_i)]$ on the observed value $g(T_i)$. Notice $1 - G_0(t) = P(C_i > t) = $ probability of a value t *not* being censored. So this scheme could be called "inverse noncensor probability" weighting.

Since $Eg(X_i) = \int g(t)dF(t)$, this expectation represents a feature of the distribution function, $F(t)$, of interest.

Notice (T_i, δ_i) is a completely observed quantity. So is Z_i. By the above lemma, the estimate/test of the mean for $Eg(X)$,

$$H_0 : Eg(X_i) = 0 \ , \tag{7.1}$$

may be translated into the new estimate/test problem for

$$H_0 : EZ_i = 0 \ . \tag{7.2}$$

However, we shall see later that this switching loses efficiency.

Since the Z_i are observed completely (no censor) and i.i.d., we can use the classic Owen [78] empirical likelihood result (our Theorem 1) to test $H_0 : EZ_i = 0$ based on i.i.d. sequence Z_i. That is, reject the null hypothesis if

$$-2\max_{p_i}\sum_{i=1}^{n}\log np_i > C$$

where the maximization over p_i is carried out for p_is such that

$$\sum_{i=1}^{n} p_i = 1, \quad \sum_{i=1}^{n} p_i Z_i = 0 \ ,$$

and C can be the chi square quantile.

There are two problems with this approach. First, the estimator based on Z_is is not an efficient estimator of $Eg(X_i)$. There is another estimator of $EZ = Eg(T_i)$ that has a smaller variance, at least asymptotically. See variance expressions in (7.3) and (7.4) below. So in the process of switching the hypothesis, we replaced the original estimating equation with a less efficient one.

The second problem is that $G_0(t)$ or $1 - G_0(t)$ is usually not available. Thus $\{Z_i\}$ are not available. We recall that $G_0(t)$ is the CDF of the censoring variables. The pseudo empirical likelihood approach tries to solve this problem by plugging in an estimator $\hat{G}(t)$, often the Kaplan–Meier estimator, and still follows Owen's classic approach. This has one consequence, that the following are no longer i.i.d. after the plug-in

$$\frac{g(T_i)\delta_i}{1 - \hat{G}(T_i)} = Z_i^*$$

since all of them involve the same estimator $\hat{G}$. Thus, Owen's classic EL approach has some difficulty when applied to $\{Z_i^*\}$.

In the analysis below, we shall assume the estimator $\hat{G}$ used in constructing $\{Z_i^*\}$ above is the Kaplan–Meier estimator $\hat{G}_{KM}(t)$. We know it is uniformly consistent for $G_0(t)$, and the mean of the (no longer i.i.d.) sequence Z_i^* is still equal to $Eg(X)$ asymptotically, but the variance of the sequence $\{Z_i^*\}$ is different from the variance of $\{Z_i\}$. In other words, $\{Z_i^*\}$ are *not* asymptotically equivalent to $\{Z_i\}$.

To be precise, we can show that, as $n \to \infty$,

$$\sqrt{n}(\bar{Z} - E(Z)) \longrightarrow N(0, \sigma_1^2) \tag{7.3}$$

and

$$\sqrt{n}(\bar{Z}^* - E(Z)) \longrightarrow N(0, \sigma_2^2) \tag{7.4}$$

in distribution, and $\sigma_1^2 > \sigma_2^2$. In the above, $\bar{Z}$ denotes the average of Z_i, etc. The above discussion also could be applied to the case where $g(t)$ is two-dimensional: $g(t) = (g_1(t), g_2(t))$ or k dimensional. Let us denote the asymptotic variance-covariance matrices of $\bar{Z}^*$ and $\bar{Z}$, when $g(t)$ is k dimensional, as

$$\Sigma_1 \quad \text{and} \quad \Sigma_2 . \tag{7.5}$$

See Srinivasan and Zhou [104] for the calculation and the expression of the two asymptotic variances or variance-covariance matrices.

We see that by plugging a Kaplan–Meier estimator for the $G_0(t)$, we improved the variance of the estimator and "solved" the $G_0(t)$ unknown problem. The only problem left is that the sequence $\{Z_i^*\}$ is no longer i.i.d. and thus the empirical likelihood of Owen [78], $\prod p_i$, is not appropriate. One indication of this fact is that the limiting distribution of Owen's log empirical likelihood ratio under the null hypothesis is no longer a chi square but a scaled chi square. See Wang and Jing [122].

Remark: The variance inequality points to the following fact: even in the unlikely event of "known $G_0(t)$," it is better to use a Kaplan–Meier estimator for the $G_0(t)$. That is, although the i.i.d. structure of Z_i makes the analysis simpler, the asymptotic variance of Z_i^* will be smaller if we instead use a Kaplan–Meier estimator to replace the *known* $G_0(t)$. See Fygenson and Zhou [31] for more discussion.

Next we examine the difference of two empirical likelihood approaches to the above test problem. Since the maximum empirical likelihood estimator and the maximum pseudo empirical likelihood estimator are identical in both approaches, that is, $\bar{Z}^* = \int g(t) d\hat{F}_{KM}(t)$ (see (7.7)), we are going to focus on the confidence regions induced by the tests.

Since for one-dimensional parameters the difference of the empirical likelihood based confidence intervals can be masked by adjusting the significance level, and for dimensions higher than three it is difficult to illustrate by plots, we focus on examples with parameters of dimension $k = 2$ later.

The pseudo empirical likelihood test uses the method developed for i.i.d. sequences, but applies it to a non-i.i.d. sequence Z_i^*. The first indication of a problem is that the limiting distribution under the null hypothesis for the pseudo empirical likelihood ratio is no longer the chi square distribution with degrees of freedom k; rather the distribution is described by a linear combination of k independent chi square df = 1 random variables.

Theorem 45 *Assume the variance of Z_i^* is finite and positive. The i.i.d. (Owen) empirical likelihood ratio based on the non-i.i.d. observations Z_i^* has the following asymptotic distribution under the null hypothesis:*

$$-2 \max_{p_i} \sum_{i=1}^{n} \log n p_i \longrightarrow \sum_{j=1}^{k} a_j \chi_{(1)j}^2$$

in distribution, where $\chi_{(1)j}^2$ $j = 1, \cdots, k$ are k independent chi square random variables with one degree of freedom, and a_j are the eigenvalues of the matrix $U = \Sigma_2 S^{-1} \Sigma_2$, with Σ_2 defined above and S the limit of sample variance matrix based on Z_i^*. The maximization in the above log EL is for all $p_i, i = 1, \cdots, n$ such that $\sum p_i = 1$, $p_i \geq 0$ $\sum p_i Z_i^* = 0$.

We refer readers to Hjort et al. [40] for the proof of this theorem.

We shall call the test based on the above procedure the pseudo empirical likelihood test. Due to the conclusion of Theorem 45, the level of significance in the pseudo empirical likelihood test can no longer be set by a simple chi square quantile, but needs to use the quantile from the CDF of the linear combination of the chi square df = 1 random variable if one wants to keep the type one error still at 5%, say.

This distribution is not only harder to work with (no table widely available, and needs estimate coefficients a_j) we argue that the confidence regions obtained by inverting the test are also sub-optimal.

In the literature, Hjort et al. [40] call this pseudo empirical likelihood a plug-in empirical likelihood, where an unknown (potentially infinite dimensional) nuisance parameter got plugged in by an estimator. They attribute the use of this approach in survival analysis to Wang and Jing [122].

7.2 Tests Based on Empirical Likelihood

To test the hypothesis

$$H_0: \ Eg(X_i) = 0$$

based on right censored data, we use the log empirical likelihood defined in (1.24), as we studied in Chapter 3. To be specific, we reject the null hypothesis if

$$-2\{\max_{w_i} \log EL_1(w_i) - \log EL_1(w_i = \Delta \hat{F}_{KM}(T_i))\} > C, \tag{7.6}$$

where the maximization over w_i is carried out for

$$\sum w_i = 1, \quad \sum w_i \delta_i g(T_i) = 0.$$

According to Chapter 3, Theorem 23, the null distribution of the above log likelihood ratio is a central chi square (a pivotal), so the constant C above can be set easily by using the quantile of chi square distribution with k degrees of freedom.

The computation of this empirical likelihood ratio is available in the package `emplik`. See Chapter 6 for a discussion of computational methods.

Remark: The two (maximum empirical likelihood) estimators in the two different empirical likelihood approaches are actually the same. The difference is in the form of the likelihood used. For any $g(\cdot)$, we have (see Chapter 5 (5.11))

$$\frac{1}{n}\sum_{i=1}^{n}\frac{g(T_i)\delta_i}{1-\hat{G}_{KM}(T_i)} = \sum_{i=1}^{n}g(T_i)\Delta\hat{F}_{KM}(T_i) . \tag{7.7}$$

So the two types of empirical likelihood achieve the maximum at the same location. The EL $\prod p_i$ achieve the maximum at $p_i = 1/n$, which gives rise to $1/n\sum Z_i^*$. This is the left-hand side of the equation above. The censored data EL, defined in Chapter 3 (6.10), achieves its maximum when $w_i = \Delta\hat{F}_{KM}(T_i)$. This gives rise to the right-hand side of the equation above.

Thus the related confidence regions are "centered" at the same point: the NPMLE.

7.3 Optimal Confidence Region

We study the confidence regions obtained by inverting the two types of test described in previous sections. We begin with a lemma concerning the confidence regions for a multivariate normal mean vector.

Lemma 46 *If an estimator $\hat{\theta}$ is multivariate normally distributed with distribution $N(\theta_0, I)$, then the confidence region for the parameter θ_0 of the type*

$$\{\theta : (\hat{\theta} - \theta)^\top(\hat{\theta} - \theta) < C\} \tag{7.8}$$

is superior when compared to the confidence regions of the type

$$\{\theta : (\hat{\theta} - \theta)^\top B(\hat{\theta} - \theta) < C^*\} \tag{7.9}$$

where B is any nonrandom, symmetric, positive definite matrix.

The optimality or superiority may be described more precisely as follows: suppose the constants C and C^* are chosen so that the two confidence regions have identical probability of covering the true parameter θ_0, then the confidence region of the first type has a smaller volume.

Remark: Obviously, if you use the matrix $B = \sigma^2 I$, then the two confidence regions will be identical. The constant σ^2 will be cancelled out when adjusting the cut off level C^*. So the lemma should be understood as "... where B is any symmetric nonnegative definite matrix other than $\sigma^2 I$ type."

PROOF: The coverage probability of the first region is

$$\int_{\|\theta_0 - \hat{\theta}\|_2 < C} f(x)dx$$

since the type I region will cover the true parameter θ_0 if and only if the L_2 distance from $\hat{\theta}$ to θ_0 is smaller than $\sqrt{C}$. In the above we denote the density of $\hat{\theta}$, $N(\theta_0, I)$, as $f(x)$.

Define a distance by $d_B(\theta_0, \hat{\theta}) = (\theta_0 - \hat{\theta})^\top B(\theta_0 - \hat{\theta})$. Then similarly the coverage probability of the second region is

$$\int_{d_B(\theta_0 - \hat{\theta}) < C^*} f(x)dx.$$

By substituting $y = \hat{\theta} - \theta_0$, we have $y \sim N(0, I)$, and the two integrals become

$$\int_{\|y\|_2 < C} f(y)dy \quad \text{and} \quad \int_{d_B(y) < C^*} f(y)dy. \tag{7.10}$$

Denote the regions of the two integrations above as R_1 and R_2. Also, let $R_1 \cap R_2 = P$. Then the requirement of equal coverage probability implies

$$\int_{R_1} f(y)dy = \int_{R_2} f(y)dy \quad \text{and} \quad \int_{R_1 \setminus P} f(y)dy = \int_{R_2 \setminus P} f(y)dy.$$

Now, the density $f(y)$ on $R_1 \setminus P$ has values at least as large as $f(y^*) = K$ for $\|y^*\|_2 = C$, since the multi-variate normal $N(0, I)$ density is a decreasing function of $\|y\|_2$.

On the other hand, the density $f(y)$ on $R_2 \setminus P$ has value at most $K = f(y^*)$. Thus

$$\int_{R_1 \setminus P} f(y)dy > \int_{R_1 \setminus P} Kdy = K \int_{R_1 \setminus P} dy = K \times vol(R_1 \setminus P)$$

and by (7.10) the left-hand side is also equal to

$$\int_{R_2 \setminus P} f(y)dy < \int_{R_2 \setminus P} Kdy = K \times vol(R_2 \setminus P).$$

Therefore, connecting the above two inequalities, we have $vol(R_2 \setminus P) > vol(R_1 \setminus P)$ and thus we also have $vol(R_2) > vol(R_1)$. It is obvious that the inequality is strict unless R_2 coincides with R_1. □

A simple linear transformation immediately gives us

Corollary 47 *In the above lemma, if $\hat{\theta}$ is normally distributed with $N(\theta_0, \Sigma)$ distribution where θ_0 is the parameter vector, then the optimal confidence region for the parameter θ_0 is*

$$\{\theta : (\hat{\theta} - \theta)^\top \Sigma^{-1}(\hat{\theta} - \theta) < C\}. \tag{7.11}$$

Remark: If the variance covariance matrix in the above lemma is only estimated consistently, then the optimality may only be asymptotic.

We claim that

(1) The confidence regions obtained by inverting an empirical likelihood ratio test (7.6) is, at least asymptotically, optimal. In other words, it is of type (7.11) or (7.8) asymptotically. This is clear from Chapter 2, Theorem 1.

(2) The confidence region obtained by inverting the pseudo empirical likelihood ratio test, even after scale adjustment, is not optimal. In fact, it is of type (7.9), asymptotically. See, for example, Hjort et al. [40].

7.4 Illustrations

We compare the confidence regions obtained by inverting the tests described above
in Figure 7.1. The larger family of regions are those obtained by inverting the pseudo
empirical likelihood tests. The smaller family of regions are those obtained by inverting the empirical likelihood ratio tests. The difference is remarkable.

It is not hard to see that when there is no censoring, the two empirical likelihood
approaches discussed above boil down to the same test, which is also the same as the
classic one studied by Owen [79]. Therefore, if $Eg(X_i)$ is not heavily influenced by
censoring, then the difference may not be too big. But in other cases, the difference
can be substantial, as the figure shows.

We took the following setting:

$$X \sim \exp(1) \quad \text{and} \quad C \sim 0.2 + \exp(1).$$

From the above X and C, we obtain T_i and δ_i via the independent random censorship
model.

The two parameters (expectations) we are going to test are

$$EX = a_1 \quad \text{and} \quad EI[X > 0.5] = a_2$$

for various constants a_1 and a_2.

From the plot, we see there is quite a difference in terms of size and orientation
between the two types of confidence regions. Next we confirm that the difference
still remains for larger samples. Fig. 7.2 is based on sample of size 2000. We see the
difference between the two types of confidence region remains.

Although the orientation and the shape difference do not necessarily show the
optimality of one type regions, they at least indicate the two types of confidence
regions are very different. What is more, the difference does not diminish as sample
size increases.

In order to definitely show the optimality of one type region, we shall try to
set the two regions at the same confidence level (90% confidence), which will then
show their area/volume difference. See Figure 7.3. According to Lemma 46, the EL
region has asymptotically smallest area among a class of regions with same coverage
probability, which includes the plug-in EL regions.

7.5 Adjustment of the Pseudo Empirical Likelihood Test

Let us call the confidence regions obtained by inverting the pseudo empirical likelihood ratio tests type I. Similarly, we call the confidence regions obtained by inverting
the empirical likelihood ratio tests type II.

Many authors, when using pseudo empirical likelihood and ending up with a
scaled chi square df = 1 distribution under the null hypothesis, suggest estimating the
scale factor and compensating for that when carrying out tests or constructing confidence intervals. After estimating the scale, the argument goes, the *inversely scaled*
pseudo empirical likelihood ratio will converge to a chi square distribution with one
degree of freedom under the null hypothesis.

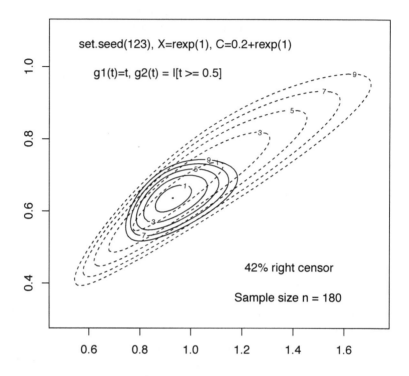

Figure 7.1: Size and shape of joint confidence regions for (a_1, a_2) from (1) EL (smaller, solid lines) and (2) plug-in EL (larger, dash lines). Sample size $n = 180$.

This is fine except the final confidence interval depends on the quality of the scale estimator and may lose the transformation invariant property if after transformation the scale becomes harder to estimate, for example. When an obvious "good" estimator of the scale exists, this is not a problem.

However, for parameters of dimension larger than two, the confidence *regions* may not be easy to scale.

To change the shape of a two-dimensional region of the type (7.9), we need a 2×2 matrix. A single constant scale can only change the relative size of the region but not its shape/orientation. Estimating this 2×2 matrix is tantamount to estimating the asymptotic variance-covariance matrix of the NPMLE.

In higher dimensions, can we recover the optimal confidence region (type II) from the confidence region of type I, after the inverse scale?

The answer is no, if we are allowed only to multiply a scale. The only way this

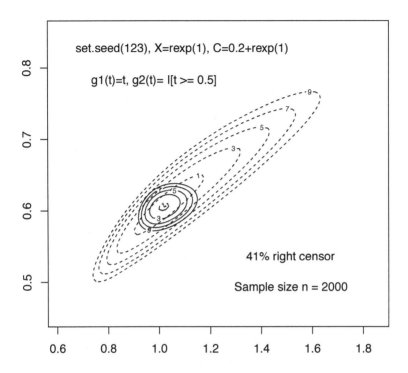

Figure 7.2: Size and shape of EL regions (smaller, solid line) and plug-in EL regions (larger, dash line). Sample size $n = 2000$. Both types of regions center at the same location.

recovery can be done (for regions of dimension larger than or equal to two) is when the multiplicative factor is (asymptotically) equal to the ratio below:

$$\frac{\log ELR(typeII)}{\log ELR(pseudo)} .$$

Obviously, this is equivalent to computing the log EL ratio (asymptotically) if not more complicated. In the literature, the estimation of $\log ELR(typeII)$ is often replaced by a quadratic form from the score test. Since asymptotically the quadratic form from the score test (or Wald test for that matter) is equivalent to the log likelihood ratio, this asymptotically will produce the "optimal region."

On the other hand, this procedure is closer to being a confidence region by inverting a score test, and probably should be called so.

Why does scaling the pseudo EL in one-dimension work? For the one-dimensional parameter, the optimal confidence intervals (asymptotically) are always symmetric intervals (due to asymptotic normality) and the scale never need to worry about that since the interval from pseudo EL is also (asymptotically) symmetric with respect to the NPMLE. For smaller sample sizes, there will be differences (e.g., skewness etc.) though.

7.6 Weighted Empirical Likelihood

Weighted empirical likelihood has been studied by many authors. In particular, Zhong and Rao [133], Wu [126], Tsao and Wu [114] used it to address the heteroscedasticity of the survey data. Ren [94], [95], however, used the weighted empirical likelihood to treat censored data inference problems. One property of the weighted empirical likelihood Ren used is that the weighted EL is maximized at the NPMLE – the Kaplan–Meier estimator. The -2 log likelihood ratio for the so defined weighted EL turns out also converging to a scaled chi square distribution.

Let us now study in more detail the weighted empirical likelihood in the right censored data situation.

Given a set of fixed weights, $w_i > 0$, define a weighted EL for the censored data (T_i, δ_i) as

$$WEL = \prod_{i=1}^{n} p_i^{w_i} ; \qquad \log WEL = \sum_{i=1}^{n} w_i \log p_i , \qquad (7.12)$$

where $p_i > 0$, $\sum_i p_i = 1$, is a probability.

Straight calculations show that when $p_i = w_i / \sum_j w_j$, the WEL achieves its maximum value. When $w_i \equiv 1$ the WEL reduces to Owen's EL for i.i.d. observations.

For a given right censored sample of observations (T_i, δ_i), let us denote the Kaplan–Meier estimator by $\hat{F}_{KM}$. Ren [94] used the weighted empirical likelihood (7.12) above with the weights $w_i = w_i^* = n \times \Delta\hat{F}_{KM}(T_i)$. (Assuming the total jumps of a Kaplan–Meier estimator is one.) Notice for this choice of weights, we have $\sum w_i = n$ and thus by design, the WEL achieves its maximum when $p_i = w_i/n = \Delta\hat{F}_{KM}(T_i)$.

Therefore, the maximum weighted empirical likelihood estimator defined this way is the same as the Kaplan–Meier estimator. Thus any confidence regions by inverting the weighted empirical likelihood ratio test will also be "centered" at the NPMLE.

However, the weighted empirical likelihood ratio test, and the induced confidence region, are different from those discussed in Chapter 3. One clue is that the null distribution of the log weighted empirical likelihood ratio is asymptotically a *scaled* chi square, not a true chi square.

The null hypothesis under consideration is the hypothesis for the mean: $Eg(X) = \mu_0$, i.e.,

$$H_0 : \sum_{i=1}^{n} g(T_i)p_i = \mu_0 .$$

If $g(\cdot) = (g_1, g_2, \cdots, g_p)$, then this is a hypothesis for p parameters. When $p_i =$

$\Delta \hat{F}_{KM}(T_i)$, $\sum g(T_i)\Delta \hat{F}_{KM}(T_i)$ is the NPMLE of $Eg(X)$. Thus the null hypothesis can also be interpreted as

$$H_0 : \int g(t)dF_x(t) = \mu_0 .$$

The test based on the weighted EL for right censored data is to reject the null hypothesis if

$$-2[\sup_{p_i} \sum_{i=1}^n w_i^* \log p_i - \sum_{i=1}^n w_i^* \log(w_i^*/n)] > C ,$$

where $w_i^* = n \times \Delta \hat{F}_{KM}(T_i)$ and the supreme is taken over all p_i such that

$$p_i \geq 0, \quad \sum_{i=1}^n p_i = 1, \quad \text{and} \quad \sum_{i=1}^n g(T_i)p_i = \mu_0 .$$

The asymptotic distribution of the log likelihood ratio test statistic under the null hypothesis has been studied by Ren [94] Theorem 3, for the case of a single parameter. We will need a multivariate version for the comparison of the confidence regions. We refer the reader to the book of Owen ([81] p. 221) for a proof in the multiple parameters case but without weights.

It is not hard to generalize the result of Owen [81] and Ren [94] to the multiple parameters weighted likelihood case. In fact, we have, under the null hypothesis H_0 above and some regularity conditions,

$$-2[\sup_{p_i} \sum_{i=1}^n w_i^* \log p_i - \sum_{i=1}^n w_i^* \log(w_i^*/n)] = U^\top V^{-1} U + o_p(1) ,$$

where

$$U = \sqrt{n}(\bar{g}_w - \mu_0) = \sqrt{n}(\frac{1}{n}\sum_{i=1}^n g(T_i)w_i^* - \mu_0)$$

and

$$V = (V_{rk}) = \frac{1}{n}\sum_{i=1}^n w_i^* (g_r(T_i) - \mu_0)(g_k(T_i) - \mu_0)^\top .$$

For the particular choice of w_i that Ren [94] proposed, $w_i = w_i^* = \Delta \hat{F}_{KM}(T_i)$, we have, under the null hypothesis,

$$U = \sqrt{n}(\int g(t)d\hat{F}_{KM}(t) - \mu_0) \xrightarrow{D} N(0, \Sigma)$$

as $n \to \infty$. For a proof of this fact and the definition of variance-covariance matrix Σ, see Lemma 21 of this book. On the other hand, an application of the law of large numbers for the Kaplan–Meier integral gives

$$V_{rk} = \int (g_r(t) - \mu_0)(g_k(t) - \mu_0)d\hat{F}_{KM}(t) \xrightarrow{P} \int (g_r(t) - \mu_0)(g_k(t) - \mu_0)dF_0(t)$$

as $n \to \infty$.

For a given set of weights, it is not hard to show that, under certain mild regularity conditions, the confidence region constructed by inverting the above weighted EL test is asymptotically equivalent to

$$\{\mu \mid (\bar{g}_w - \mu)\Sigma_w^{-1}(\bar{g}_w - \mu)^\top < C\} ,$$

where $\bar{g}_w$ is the weighted average of the $g(T_i)$s:

$$\bar{g}_w = \frac{1}{n}\sum_{i=1}^{n} g(T_i)w_i^*$$

and Σ_w is the sample variance and covariance matrix from the weighted sample:

$$\sum w_i^* w_j^* (g(T_i) - \bar{g}_w)(g(T_j) - \bar{g}_w)^\top .$$

In view of Hjort et al. ([40] Theorem 2.1) and our Corollary 47, we have the following.

Lemma 48 *The above weighted empirical likelihood confidence interval will be asymptotically optimal (in the sense we discussed in the previous section) if and only if the asymptotic variance-covariance of the mean estimator*

$$\hat{\mu} = \int g(t)d\hat{F}_{KM}(t) = \sum g(T_i)w_i^*$$

can be consistently estimated by

$$\int (g_r(t) - \mu_0)(g_k(t) - \mu_0)^\top d\hat{F}_{KM}(t) . \qquad (7.13)$$

Obviously, the true asymptotic variance of $\hat{\mu}$ is more complicated than (7.13). For one thing, we know the true asymptotic variance-covariance of the Kaplan–Meier integral depends on the censoring distribution $G_0(t)$, but the limit of (7.13) is free from G_0. Therefore, the confidence region obtained by inverting the weighted empirical likelihood ratio test above is not optimal.

This confidence region obviously also suffers from the same drawback as the plug-in empirical likelihood because the variance-covariance matrix is not the right one as required by our Lemma 46. If the data were independent with no censoring, and the weight represents the (inverse of) variance of each observation, then the sample variance-covariance matrix would be correct, and the confidence region would be optimal.

The following plot (Fig. 7.3) is based on a right censored sample of size $n = 1000$. It shows the three 90% confidence regions from inverting (1) the EL test we discussed in Chapter 3, (2) the plug-in EL test, and (3) the weighted EL test just discussed.

We notice that all three regions center at the same spot, which is the NPMLE value. But the shape and size of the regions are quite different. Recall from the discussion in Section 7.3 that the confidence region from the EL test is optimal, at least asymptotically.

In order to get a fair comparison, we have set the level of the confidence for the

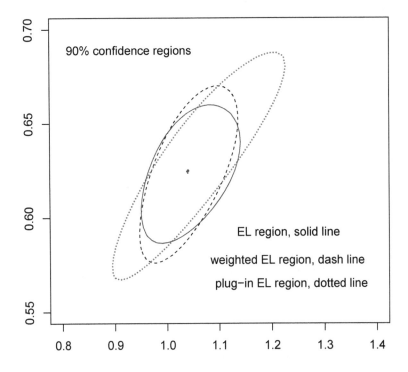

Figure 7.3: Three confidence regions by (1) EL (solid line, smallest volume), (2) plug-in EL (dotted line, largest volume) and (3) weighted EL (dash line). The three contours have same center.

three regions by using simulation: we simulated each of the three tests under the null hypothesis 10,000 times and took the sample 90th percentile of the empirical distributions of the three test statistics as our critical values.

The difference in the three confidence regions will diminish when the censoring percentage dwindles to zero. But the sample size increment does not make the confidence regions closer to each other.

Remark: Zhou [138] proposed an iteration scheme (EM algorithm) with censored data by weighted empirical likelihood. In particular, he showed that if we use the jumps of the *constrained* Kaplan–Meier estimator as the weights, the iteration procedure will converge because it is a type of EM algorithm. The converged limiting CDF is none other than the constrained NPMLE for censored data. The constrained NPMLE or constrained Kaplan–Meier estimator was then used to construct the censored empirical likelihood ratio.

In addition to the difference in the definition of the EL, a closer examination reveals that the constrained NPMLE of Ren's weighted EL is equivalent to Zhou's [138] but stopped at iteration one.

7.6.1   A Final Comment

The plug-in empirical likelihood often makes mathematical analysis easier and computations simpler. But this is achieved at the cost of (1) possible loss of optimality when constructing confidence regions, (2) harder to set the significance level of the resulting test, or the confidence level, due to complicated null distribution.

On the other hand, when our primary goal is to obtain confidence intervals/testing of a *single parameter* instead of confidence regions or testing multiple parameters, the adjusted plug-in empirical likelihood could work similarly to the empirical likelihood for large samples, provided, of course, the correct adjustment is used in view of the scaled chi square degree of freedom one distribution.

It is not clear if the adjusted plug-in empirical likelihood ratio test maintains the transformation invariance property of the likelihood ratio test or not (depends on the scale estimator). Also, for smaller sample sizes, the confidence intervals from plug-in empirical likelihood (even after adjustment) can be quite different from those obtained from the empirical likelihood. The main difference is whether the intervals are symmetric or not.

7.7   Discussion and Historic Notes

We have not discussed the higher order asymptotic property of the empirical likelihood ratio in this book. In particular, we did not look at the possibility of Bartlett corrections or bootstrap calibrations.

Kitamura [56] and Kitamura et al. [58] also studied the optimality of the empirical likelihood test via its asymptotic type I and type II errors. But the shape difference of the confidence regions seems more dramatic and reveals the important link between the chi square limit under the null hypothesis and correct shape and orientation of the confidence region. See Kim and Zhou [54].

We have restricted our discussion to the family of confidence regions of type $\{\theta | (\hat{\theta} - \theta)^\top B(\hat{\theta} - \theta) < C\}$. Outside this restriction, it is known that you can have better confidence regions for high dimensional normal mean parameters (Stein phenomena). See Efron [23] for details.

Chapter 8

Miscellaneous

In this chapter we discuss some topics that do not belong in any of the previous chapters. In particular we collect several confidence band constructions by empirical likelihood.

8.1 Smoothing

In the study of the empirical likelihood ratio test for quantiles, if we plot the EL against the quantiles (similar to Figure 3.2), it will be obvious that some smoothing can help improve chi square approximations.

Indeed, any statistics that have to do with quantiles can benefit from smoothing. This includes (1) medians and quantiles of survival probabilities, (2) trimmed means since the trimming proportion has to do with quantiles and (3) (generalized) Lorenz curves.

Chen and Hall [12] proposed and studied a class of smoothing method and concluded that smoothing can improve the chi square approximation for the EL test for quantile to $O(1/n)$ error under the null hypothesis. We expect the same rate of improvement to hold with censored data empirical likelihood ratios. Chen and Hall [12] also studied further improvement using Edgeworth expansions.

Another place where smoothing may be useful is where ranks of the data are used to define the statistics of interest, for example, the rank estimator of the AFT model we discussed in Chapters 2 and 5. Heller [38] proposed a type of smoothing and found the rank-based estimating equation is easier to solve after smoothing, yet it preserves the asymptotic distribution of the estimator produced. This smoothing should also help improve the chi square approximation for the EL test.

We have not explored smoothing in this book. No smoothing is included in the package emplik.

8.2 Exponential Tilted Likelihood

The proposal to use an exponential function to tilt the original equal weights of EL for observed data appears to have been first proposed in the context of the bootstrap [19]. In the empirical likelihood for i.i.d data, the equal probability of $1/n$ from the empirical distribution can also be tilted using the exponential function. Owen [81] includes some discussion about this. See also Jing and Wood [48]. But it seems that the use of exponential tilted empirical likelihood is only limited to uncensored data. It is not clear how one should modify the exponentially tilted empirical likelihood ratio to handle right censored data. So we shall be satisfied with a brief introduction here.

In this section, the sample is a noncensored i.i.d. observation $X_1, X_2, \cdots, X_n$. Define a family of distribution functions that are dominated by the empirical distribution function, and the point mass placed on the ith observation X_i is given by

$$p_i = p_i(t) = \frac{\exp(t(X_i - \mu))}{\sum_{j=1}^{n} \exp(t(X_j - \mu))} , \tag{8.1}$$

where t is the so-called tilting parameter and μ is the direction of the tilt. Clearly, when $t = 0$, we have $p_i = 1/n$, which corresponds to the empirical distribution as a special case. For $t \neq 0$, the defined p_i is *always* a probability, due to the fact that exponential functions are always positive. With the tilted exponential weights, the weighted mean is

$$\mu(t) = \sum_i X_i p_i(t) = \sum_{i=1}^{n} X_i \frac{\exp(t(X_i - \mu))}{\sum_{j=1}^{n} \exp(t(X_j - \mu))} .$$

Remark: The above distribution family is indexed by t and it plays a similar role as the λ in formula (1.17). But not all λ values give rise to a probability in (1.17).

For $t \neq 0$, the above p_i will induce a distribution with a mean value depending on t (and different from the sample mean). Adjusting t to satisfy the null hypothesis gives rise to a distribution satisfying H_0.

It has been shown that exponential tilted empirical likelihood is equivalent to regular empirical likelihood in the first order (up to order $o(1)$) in the noncensored case. We point out that this is due to the similarity of the Taylor expansion of the two probabilities at $t = 0$:

$$n \times p_i(t) = 1 + tA - \frac{1}{2}t^2 A^2 + \cdots ;$$

and (from 1.17)

$$n \times p_i(\lambda) = 1 + \lambda A .$$

However, for higher order properties, the exponentially tilted empirical likelihood does not seem to work as well as the regularly tilted probabilities. See Jing and Wood [48].

The advantage of the exponential tilting likelihood is that for *any* t, the defined probability $p_i(t)$ in (8.1) is always between 0 and 1 and sums to 1. So there is no feasibility problem. For the regular empirical likelihood (1.17), the tilted probability is given by (normalization if needed)

$$p_i(\lambda) = \frac{1}{n + \lambda(X_i - \mu)} ,$$

which is easy to see that, only for λ in a neighborhood around zero, the defined p_i are between 0 and 1. In fact, for certain values of λ, p_i can approach infinity or become negative. And the neighborhood depends on the observed data X_i and μ. We term these the feasible values when discussing them in Chapter 1 and 2.

When tilted empirical likelihoods are needed for a large domain of the tilting parameter λ, this can be a problem. For example, when using empirical likelihood to carry out Bayesian type analysis, it will be easier to define a prior for λ if λ is allowed to vary on the whole line.

We shall not discuss the possible use of empirical likelihood in Bayesian analysis here, but refer readers to Lazard [65], Mergersen et al. [72] and Schennach [100], [101].

For empirical likelihood tests under the null hypothesis or under local alternatives, we still prefer the regular empirical likelihood tilting due to its optimality property (constrained NPMLE). Another possibility to handle infinite or negative p_i in the above definition is to modify the logarithm function near zero and on the negative domain, so that for zero or negative values, it is still well defined instead of returning an infinite or undefined. This is in fact how Owen's original S-plus code elm( ) handles the possibility of NA in log EL. We have followed his approach in emplik.

For censored data empirical likelihood analysis, it is conceivable that we can try an exponentially tilted hazard function empirical likelihood in the context of Chapter 1. But it is not clear if an exponential tilt will work for the censored empirical likelihood in terms of the CDF.

8.3   Confidence Bands

Confidence bands or simultaneous confidence intervals provide a global picture about a function over time. A 95% confidence band for a survival function over $[a,b]$, for example, is supposed to cover the true survival curve for all $t \in [a,b]$ entirely with 95% probability. A confidence interval for survival probability at a time t_0 is just a confidence band with $a = b = t_0$.

Empirical likelihood can also be used to construct a confidence band. However, there is no clear criteria for an optimal confidence band.

A confidence band can be viewed as a rectangular confidence region with infinitely many sides. Even for a rectangular confidence region of two sides (for two parameters), no optimality can be easily formulated, since one may sacrifice one side to improve the other side in a variety of ways. Therefore, when we discuss confidence bands, the optimality properties like those discussed in Chapter 7 are off. Nevertheless, the band based on EL is transformation invariant, range respecting and generally a good choice compared to other available methods, as many simulations show. Roughly speaking, an empirical likelihood ratio confidence band is similar to the Wald confidence band provided we apply possibly different transformations to different $t \in [a,b]$.

The confidence bands we shall discuss below all have the so-called "equal-precision" property: suppose $[L(t), U(t)]$ is a 95% confidence band for a true function

$g(t)$ over $t \in [a,b]$; then for any fixed $t \in [a,b]$ the probability $P(L(t) \leq g(t) \leq U(t))$ does not depend on t and should be higher than 0.95.

For a fixed t, the confidence interval for $g(t)$ can be constructed using EL, as we discussed in previous chapters.

(1) For $g(t)$ as survival probability at t or cumulative hazard at t, see Examples 8, 14, 25, 29.

(2) For $g(t)$ as the ratio of two survival probabilities at t, see Exercise 3.2 but also see Example 16, which is for the ratio $F_1(t)/F_2(t)$.

(3) For $g(t)$ as the ratio of two cumulative hazards, see Example 31.

(4) For $g(t)$ as the difference of two survival functions, see Example 16.

(5) For $g(t)$ as the cumulative hazard within a Cox model, see Example 20.

In order to obtain the confidence band, we need to replace the significance threshold in constructing the point-wise confidence interval with a larger value. For example, for a 95% confidence interval we used 3.84 as the threshold value for the log EL ratio. Now 3.84 needs to be replaced by a larger value when constructing a confidence band over $t \in [a,b]$. Once we do that, repeatedly constructing confidence intervals (using this inflated threshold value) for all $t \in [a,b]$ will give the band.

The exact value of this inflated threshold depends on $[a,b]$ and on the underlying $g(t)$, etc. So constructing a table for every situation is not feasible. In practice we use simulation to find this constant, for given $[a,b]$ and estimated $\hat{g}(t)$, etc., based on the limiting process of the log EL ratio, which we shall discuss in detail below.

8.3.1   One Sample

For fixed time t, denote the empirical likelihood test of $H_0 : S(t) = \theta(t)$ (where $S(t) = 1 - F(t)$ is the survival function) as

$$-2\log ELR(\theta(t),t) .$$

We have done such examples in Chapter 3 and know the null distribution of the test is asymptotically chi square with one degree of freedom. Now we shall consider t as a variable and view the above test statistic as a process in t.

Hollander et al. [41] have shown that as n increases, this process converges in $D[a,b]$ in distribution to a limiting process that can be described as

$$\left[\frac{B(\sigma^2(t))}{\sigma(t)} \right]^2 \tag{8.2}$$

where

$$\sigma^2(t) = \int_0^t \frac{d\Lambda(s)}{[1 - F(s-)][1 - G(s-)]},$$

and $B(\cdot)$ is a Brownian motion.

Therefore, let C be a constant such that

$$P\left(\sup_{a \leq t \leq b} \left[\frac{B(\sigma^2(t))}{\sigma(t)} \right]^2 < C \right) = 0.9 .$$

Then a 90% confidence band for the survival curve $S(t)$ over $[a,b]$ can be obtained as

$$\{(\theta(t),t);\ t \in [a,b] \mid -2\log ELR(\theta(t),t) < C\}\ .$$

8.3.2 Two Independent Samples

There are several ways we can compare the two-sample survival/hazard functions.

1. Ratio of two survival functions. By taking a log function, this immediately becomes a band for the difference of two cumulative hazard functions.

McKeague and Zhao [71] studied the limiting behavior of the log EL ratio as a process. They show the log EL ratio process converges in $D[a,b]$ to a limiting process. The limiting process can be described by

$$\left[\frac{B(\sigma^2(t))}{\sigma(t)}\right]^2 \tag{8.3}$$

where

$$\sigma^2(t) = \frac{1}{p_1}\int_0^t \frac{d\Lambda_1(s)}{[1-F_1(s-)][1-G_1(s-)]} + \frac{1}{p_2}\int_0^t \frac{d\Lambda_2(s)}{[1-F_2(s-)][1-G_2(s-)]}$$

where $p_i = \lim n_i/(n_1 + n_2)$ is the proportion of each sample size to the total, and $B(t)$ is a standard Brownian motion.

We notice that the process at any fixed time t is a chi square distribution with one degree of freedom.

2. Difference of two survival functions. Shen and He [103] studied the limiting behavior of the log EL ratio in this situation. Similar to the above, they show the limiting process for the log empirical likelihood ratio is

$$\left[\frac{U(t)}{\sigma(t)}\right]^2 \tag{8.4}$$

where

$$U(t) = \frac{[S_1(t)]B_1(\sigma_1^2(t))}{\sqrt{p_1}} + \frac{S_2(t)B_2(\sigma_2^2(t))}{\sqrt{p_2}}\ ,$$

$B_1(t)$ and $B_2(t)$ are two independent Brownian motions and

$$\sigma_i^2(t) = \int_0^t \frac{d\Lambda_i(s)}{[1-F_i(s-)][1-G_i(s-)]}\ ,\qquad i = 1,2.$$

Finally, we have

$$\sigma^2(t) = \mathrm{Var}[U(t)]\ .$$

This also imply that the process in (8.4) has the property that for fixed time t, it is a chi square distribution with one degree of freedom.

8.3.3   Band within a Cox Model

For Cox models with a single baseline hazard function, we have discussed how to construct a confidence band of baseline survival by empirical likelihood in Chapter 4, Section 4.3.

For stratified Cox models with two (or more) baseline hazard functions, the confidence band for the ratio of the two baselines was considered by Wei and Schaubel [123] and Dong and Matthews [22]. Zhu et al. [147] showed how to construct an EL based confidence band for the ratio of the two baseline cumulative hazards while adjusting for covariates.

Define the log EL for a stratified Cox model with two arbitrary baseline functions as follows:

$$\log EL(\beta, p) = \sum_{i=1}^{2} \sum_{j=1}^{n_i} \{p_{ij} \exp(z_{ij}\beta)\}^{\delta_{ij}} \exp\{-\exp(z_{ij}\beta) \sum_{k=1}^{n_i} I[T_{ik} \le T_{ij}] p_{ij}\}.$$

This log EL is maximized when β equals to the Cox partial likelihood estimator, and p_{ij} equals the jump of the Breslow baseline estimator.

To test the null hypothesis

$$H_0 : \Lambda_{01}(t)/\Lambda_{02}(t) = \theta_0(t) ,$$

we need also to find the maximum of the log EL under constraint

$$\sum_{j=1}^{n_1} p_{1j} I[T_{1j} \le t] = \theta(t) \sum_{j=1}^{n_2} p_{2j} I[T_{2j} \le t]$$

while holding β equal to the Cox partial likelihood estimator. Two times the difference of the unconstrained and constrained maximum log EL will be our test statistic. Let us denote the test statistic by $-2\log ELR(\theta_0(t), t)$.

Zhu et al. [147] show that under the null hypothesis $-2\log ELR(\theta_0(t), t)$ converge as a process in $D[a, b]$ to a limiting process. The limiting distribution of the log EL ratio process under the null hypothesis can be characterized by

$$\frac{U^2(t)}{\sigma^2(t)} ,$$

where U is a mean zero Gaussian process with variance-covariance function $v(t, s)$ and

$$h_i(t) = \int_0^t z_i^{(1)}(\beta_0, u)/z_i^{(0)}(\beta_0, u) d\Lambda_i(u), \quad i = 1, 2,$$

$$\sigma^2(t) = \int_0^t d\Lambda_1(u)/z_1^{(0)}(\beta_0, u) + \theta_0^2(t) \int_0^t d\Lambda_2(u)/z_2^{(0)}(\beta_0, u), \quad (8.5)$$

$$v(t, s) = \sigma^2(t \wedge s) + \{h_1(s) - \theta_0(s)h_2(s)\}^\top \Sigma^{-1} \{h_1(t) - \theta_0(t)h_2(t)\},$$

where Σ is the Cox information matrix for the parameter β, and $z^{(0)}, z^{(1)}$ are the the weighted covariate processes defined in Chapter 4. Finally, $\theta(t)$ here is the ratio of two cumulative hazards.

In all the above construction of the confidence bands, we always need to find the threshold constant C, and usually this has to be done by simulation. The Gaussian process involved in the one- and two-sample cases have independent increments, while in the Cox model setting, it does not. In our experience, the simulation is pretty fast and only needs the random generation of normal random variables (in addition to the sample data) even for the nonindependent increment case.

The variance function $\sigma^2(t)$ in each case above appearing in the limiting processes needs to be estimated. In all the cases above, the estimator is obtained by replacing $\Lambda(t)$ with $\hat{\Lambda}_{NA}(t)$, etc. The resulting estimator is a piecewise constant function, say $\hat{\sigma}^2(t)$, which is uniformly and strongly consistent. It is very easy to simulate $B(\hat{\sigma}^2(t))$ by using the piecewise constant property of $\hat{\sigma}^2(t)$: it is just a summation of a series of independent normal random variables. Each jump of the $\hat{\sigma}^2(t)$ function corresponds to a normal random variable in the summation.

Zhu et al. [147] also includes several simulation studies where the just discussed estimation method was applied and final confidence band is illustrated.

The confidence band we study in Chapter 3 is also for the cumulative baseline hazard in the Cox model. Compared to the Lin et al. [69] procedure, we see some differences.

Our confidence band is based on the empirical likelihood ratio, and thus no explicit transformation is needed when calculating the confidence band. On the other hand, some transformation, often log-log, is needed for the Lin et al. [69] procedure since they use normal approximation in the construction of the band. This problem is more profound when we are dealing with the difference of two survival functions. It is impossible to apply log-log transformation to $S_1(t) - S_2(t)$, and what other transformation to use is not clear. When a confidence band over a wide interval $[a, b]$ is constructed by the normal approximation method, the appropriate transformation for t near the right end b may be different from those required by t near left end a. In other words, the appropriate choice of transformation is t dependent. It is not easy to transition from one transformation to the other when t varies in $[a, b]$. Empirical likelihood based confidence bands do not need to worry about transformations.

The computation software, however, is not yet included in the R package. More development is needed before the code is robust enough for public consumption.

8.4   Discussion and Historic Notes

Smoothing is a topic that has a huge list of literature. The smoothing methods used by Chen and Hall [12] and Heller [38] both try to replace an indicator function by a smooth function in the definition of the estimator/estimating equation. Another possibility is to leave the estimating equation unchanged and directly smooth the EL value. This method has the advantage of leaving the NPMLE unchanged before and after the smoothing, if the smoothing is done properly.

Confidence bands were considered by many authors, but most of them did not use empirical likelihood. Owen [81] includes a chapter on bands but does not treat censored data. Parzen et al. [85], Zhang and Klein [132] and Wei and Schaubel [123] considered confidence bands inside a Cox model.

Some earlier references for different types of confidence bands include Bie et al. [9], and in a two-sample setting, Dabrowska et al. [18]. For a comparison of the bands, see Nair [77].

For stratified Cox models, if our interest is in the difference of two individualized survival functions from two strata, a similar construction of the log EL to Section 8.3.3 can be used. In fact, Zhu [145] includes a result on the limiting process of the test statistic and several examples.

We have not included any procedures that construct confidence bands for the quantiles or Q–Q plots. For those, please see Hollander et al. [42] and Einmahl and McKeague [25].

We have not discussed the higher order asymptotic property of the empirical likelihood ratio in this book. In particular, we did not look at the possibility of Bartlett correction. We also did not touch the topic of more complicated censoring, where EL can be very useful.

8.5 Exercise

Exercise 8.1 *For two independent right censored samples, test the hypothesis (for any fixed τ and given η_τ, $\theta(\tau)$)*

$$H_{00} : \Lambda_1(\tau) = \eta_\tau, \ \Lambda_2(\tau) = \theta(\tau)\eta_\tau ,$$

using the empirical likelihood ratio.

Denote the empirical likelihood ratio for testing the above hypothesis as

$$-2\log ELR(\eta_\tau, \theta(\tau), \tau) .$$

Show that the above test statistic converges in distribution to a chi square degree of freedom two distribution when the η and θ values are the true values.

Next, find the η_τ value that minimizes the test statistic. Denote the maximizer by $\hat{\eta}_\tau$.

Finally, assume the $\theta(t)$ is the true value of the ratio $\Lambda_2(t)/\Lambda_1(t)$, show that for $t \in [a,b]$ the test statistic, as a process in $D[a,b]$,

$$-2\log ELR(\hat{\eta}_t, \theta(t), t) ,$$

converges in distribution to a limit. Identify the limiting process.

References

[1] O. Aalen. Nonparametric inference for a family of counting processes. *Annals of Statistics*, 6:701–726, 1978.

[2] M. Akritas. The central limit theorem under censoring. *Bernoulli*, 6:1109–1120, 2000.

[3] P. K. Andersen, Ø. Borgan, R. Gill, and N. Keiding. *Statistical Models Based on Counting Processes*. Springer, 1993.

[4] P. K. Andersen and R. D. Gill. Cox's regression model for counting processes: a large sample study. *Annals of Statistics*, 10(4):1100–1120, 1982.

[5] W. Barton. *Comparison of Two Samples by a Nonparametric Likelihood-Ratio Test*. Ph.D. Dissertation, University of Kentucky, 2010.

[6] A. Bathke, M. Kim, and M. Zhou. Combined multiple testing by censored empirical likelihood. *Journal of Statistical Planning and Inference*, 139:814–827, 2009.

[7] C. Beach and R. Davidson. Distribution-free statistical inference with Lorenz curves and income shares. *Review of Economic Studies*, 50:723–735, 1983.

[8] P. Bickel, C. Klaassen, Y. Ritov, and J. Wellner. *Efficient and Adaptive Estimation for Semiparametric Models*. Springer, 1998.

[9] O. Bie, Ø. Borgan, and K. Liestøl. Confidence intervals and confidence bands for the cumulative hazard rate function and their small sample properties. *Scandinavian Journal of Statistics*, pages 221–233, 1987.

[10] J. J. Buckley and I. R. James. Linear regression with censored data. *Biometrika*, 66:429–436, 1979.

[11] S. Chakraborti. Asymptotically distribution-free joint confidence intervals for generalized Lorenz curves based on complete data. *Statistics and Probability Letters*, 21:229–235, 1994.

[12] S. Chen and P. Hall. Smoothed empirical likelihood confidence intervals for quantiles. *Annals of Statistics*, 21:1166–1181, 1993.

[13] X. Chen and H. Cui. Empirical likelihood inference for partial linear models under martingale difference sequence. *Statistics and Probability Letters*, 78:2895–2901, 2008.

[14] F. Cowell and M. Victoria-Feser. Statistical inference for Lorenz curves with censored data. Discussion Paper No. DARP 35, 1998.

[15] D. R. Cox. Regression models and life-tables. *Journal of the Royal Statistical*

Society. Series B (Methodological), pages 187–220, 1972.

[16] D. R. Cox. Partial likelihood. *Biometrika*, 62(2):269–276, 1975.

[17] I. D. Currie. A note on Buckley–James estimators for censored data. *Biometrika*, 83:912–915, 1996.

[18] D. Dabrowska, K. Doksum, and J. Song. Graphical comparison of cumulative hazards for two populations. *Biometrika*, 76(4):763–773, 1989.

[19] A. C. Davison and D. V. Hinkley. *Bootstrap Methods and Their Application*. Cambridge University Press, 1997.

[20] G. Diao, D. Zeng, and S. Yang. Efficient semiparametric estimation of short-term and long-term hazard ratios with right-censored data. *Biometrics*, 69:840–849, 2013.

[21] T. DiCiccio, P. Hall, and J. Romano. Empirical likelihood is Bartlett-correctable. *Annals of Statistics*, 19:1053–1061, 1991.

[22] B. Dong and D. Matthews. Empirical likelihood for cumulative hazard ratio estimation with covariate adjustment. *Biometrics*, 68(2):408–418, 2012.

[23] B. Efron. Minimum volume confidence regions for a multivariate normal mean vector. *Journal of the Royal Statistical Society: Series B*, 68:655–670, 2006.

[24] B. Efron and I. M. Johnstone. Fisher's information in terms of the hazard rate. *Annals of Statistics*, 18:38–62, 1990.

[25] J. Einmahl and I. McKeague. Confidence tubes for multiple quantile plots via empirical likelihood. *Annals of Statistics*, 27(4):1348–1367, 1999.

[26] H. Fang. *Binomial Empirical Likelihood Ratio Method in Survival Analysis*. Ph.D. Dissertation, University of Kentucky, 2000.

[27] D. Finkelstein, A. Muzikansky, and D. Schoenfeld. Comparing survival of a sample to that of a standard population. *Journal of the National Cancer Institute*, 95:1434–1439, 2003.

[28] T. R. Fleming and D. P. Harrington. *Counting Process and Survival Analysis*. John Wiley, New York, 1991.

[29] D. A. Freedman. Bootstrapping regression models. *Annals of Statistics*, 9:1218–1228, 1981.

[30] M. Fygenson and Y. Ritov. Monotone estimating equations for censored data. *Annals of Statistics*, 22:732–746, 1994.

[31] M. Fygenson and M. Zhou. On using stratification in the analysis of linear regression models with right censoring. *Annals of Statistics*, 22:747–762, 1994.

[32] J. L. Gastwirth. The estimation of the Lorenz curve and Gini index. *Review of Economics and Statistics*, 54:306–316, 1972.

[33] D. P. Gaver and R. G. Miller. Jackknifing the Kaplan–Meier survival estimator for censored data: Simulation results and asymptotic analysis. *Commun. in Statis. A*, 12:1701–1718, 1983.

[34] C. Gigliarano and P. Muliere. Estimating the Lorenz curve and Gini index with right censored data: A Polya tree approach. *Metron*, 71:105–122, 2013.

[35] R. Gill. *Censoring and Stochastic Integrals*. Mathematisch Centrum track 124, 1980.

[36] R. Gill. Large sample behaviour of the product-limit estimator on the whole line. *Annals of Statistics*, 11:49–58, 1983.

[37] S. Gross and T. L. Lai. Nonparametric estimation and regression analysis with left truncated and right censored data. *Journal of the American Statistical Association*, 91:1166–1180, 1996.

[38] G. Heller. Smoothed rank regression with censored data. *Journal of the American Statistical Association*, 102:552–559, 2007.

[39] G. Heller and J. Simonoff. Prediction in censored survival data: A comparison of the proportional hazards and linear regression models. *Biometrics*, 48:101–115, 1992.

[40] N. L. Hjort, I. McKeague, and I. V. Keilegom. Extending the scope of empirical likelihood. *Annals of Statistics*, 37:1079–1111, 2009.

[41] M. Hollander, I. McKeague, and J. Yang. Likelihood ratio based confidence bands for survival functions. *Journal of American Statistical Association*, 92:215–226, 1997.

[42] M. Hollander, I. McKeague, J. Yang, and G. Li. Nonparametric likelihood ratio confidence bands for quantile functions from incomplete survival data. *Annals of Statistics*, 24:628–640, 1996.

[43] Y. Hu. *Some contributions to the censored empirical likelihood with hazard-type constraints*. Ph.D. Dissertation, University of Kentucky, 2011.

[44] Y. Hu and M. Zhou. Hazard estimating equations and empirical likelihood. Tech Report, University of Kentucky, 2013.

[45] J. Huang, S. Ma, and H. Xie. Least absolute deviations estimation for the accelerated failure time model. *Statistica Sinica*, 17:1533–1548, 2007.

[46] J. Jeong, S. H. Jung, and J. P. Costantino. Nonparametric inference on median residual life function. *Biometrics*, 64:157–163, 2008.

[47] Z. Jin, D. Y. Lin, L. J. Wei, and Z. Ying. Rank-based inference for the accelerated failure time model. *Biometrika*, 90:341–353, 2003.

[48] B. Jing and A. Wood. Exponential empirical likelihood is not Bartlett correctable. *Annals of Statistics*, 24:365–369, 1996.

[49] B. Jing, J. Yuan, and W. Zhou. Jackknife empirical likelihood. *Journal of the American Statistical Association*, 104:1224–1232, 2009.

[50] S. Johansen. An extension of Cox's regression model. *International Statistical Review/Revue Internationale de Statistique*, pages 165–174, 1983.

[51] J. Kalbfleisch and R. Prentice. *The Statistical Analysis of Failure Time Data, 2nd ed.* Wiley, 2002.

[52] E. L. Kaplan and P. Meier. Nonparametric estimation from incomplete observations. *Journal of the American Statistical Association*, 53(282):457–481,
1958.

[53] J. Kiefer and J. Wolfowitz. Consistency of the maximum likelihood estimator
in the presence of infinitely many incidental parameters. *Annals of Mathematical Statistics*, 27(4):887–906, 1956.

[54] M. Kim and M. Zhou. Comparison of extended empirical likelihood methods:
Size and shape of confidence regions from extended empirical likelihood tests.
Tech Report, University of Kentucky, 2014.

[55] M. Kim, M. Zhou, and J. Jeong. Censored quantile regression for residual
lifetimes. *Lifetime Data Analysis*, 18:177–194, 2012.

[56] Y. Kitamura. Asymptotic optimality of empirical likelihood for testing moment restrictions. *Econometrca*, 69:369–401, 2001.

[57] Y. Kitamura. Empirical likelihood methods in econometrics: Theory and practice. In *Advances in Economics and Econometrics: Theory and Applications,
Ninth World Congress,* ed. by R. Blundell, W. K. Newey, and T. Persson. Cambridge University Press, 2006.

[58] Y. Kitamura, A. Santos, and A. M. Shaikh. On the asymptotic optimality of
empirical likelihood for testing moment restrictions. *Econometrca*, 80:413–
423, 2012.

[59] J. P. Klein and M. L. Moeschberger. *Survival Analysis, Techniques for Censored and Truncated Data.* Springer, 2nd edition, 2003.

[60] R. Koenker. *Quantile Regression.* Cambridge University Press, 2005.

[61] R. Koenker and G. Basset. Regression quantiles. *Econometrika*, 46:33–50,
1978.

[62] H. Koul, V. Susarla, and J. Van Ryzin. Regression analysis with randomly
right-censored data. *Annals of Statistics*, 9:1276–1288, 1981.

[63] H. Koul, V. Susarla, and J. Van Ryzin. Least squares regression analysis with
censored survival data. In *Topics in Applied Statistics,* Ed. Y. P. Chaubey and
T. D. Dwivedi; Marcel Dekker New York, pages 151–165, 1982.

[64] T. L. Lai and Z. Ying. Large sample theory of a modified Buckley–James
estimator for regression analysis with censored data. *Annals of Statistics*,
19:1370–1402, 1991.

[65] N. Lazar. Bayesian empirical likelihood. *Biometrika*, 90:319–326, 2003.

[66] S. Leurgans. Linear models, random censoring and synthetic data. *Biometrika*,
74:301–309, 1987.

[67] G. Li. On nonparametric likelihood ratio estimation of survival probabilities
for censored data. *Statistics and Probability Letters*, 25(2):95–104, 1995.

[68] G. Li, R. Li, and M. Zhou. Empirical likelihood in survival analysis. In
Contemporary Multivariate Analysis and Design of Experiments, Edited by J.
Fan and G. Li; World Scientific Publisher, pages 337–350, 2005.

[69] D. Y. Lin, T. R. Fleming, and L. J. Wei. Confidence bands for survival curves under the proportional hazards model. *Biometrika*, 81(1):73–81, 1994.

[70] J. S. Lin and L. J. Wei. Linear regression analysis based on Buckley–James estimating equations. *Biometrics*, 48:679–681, 1992.

[71] I. McKeague and Y. Zhao. Simultaneous confidence bands for ratios of survival functions via empirical likelihood. *Statistics and Probability Letters*, 60:405–415, 2002.

[72] K. Mergersen, P. Pudlo, and C. Robert. Bayesian computation via empirical likelihood. *Proceedings of the National Academy of Sciences*, 110:1321–1326, 2012.

[73] R. Miller and J. Halpern. Regression with censored data. *Biometrika*, 69:521–531, 1982.

[74] S. A. Murphy. Likelihood ratio-based confidence intervals in survival analysis. *Journal of the American Statistical Association*, 90(432):1399–1405, 1995.

[75] S. A. Murphy and A. W. van der Vaart. Semiparametric likelihood ratio inference. *Annals of Statistics*, 25:1471–1509, 1997.

[76] U. V. Naik-Nimbalkar and M. B. Rajarshi. Empirical likelihood ratio test for equality of k medians in censored data. *Statistics and Probability Letters*, 34:267–273, 1997.

[77] V. N. Nair. Confidence bands for survival functions with censored data: A comparative study. *Technometrics*, 26(3):265–275, 1984.

[78] A. B. Owen. Empirical likelihood ratio confidence intervals for a single functional. *Biometrika*, 75(2):237–249, 1988.

[79] A. B. Owen. Empirical likelihood confidence regions. *Annals of Statistics*, 18:90–120, 1990.

[80] A. B. Owen. Empirical likelihood for linear models. *Annals of Statistics*, 19:1725–1747, 1991.

[81] A. B. Owen. *Empirical Likelihood*. CRC Press, 2001.

[82] A. B. Owen. Self-concordance for empirical likelihood. *Canadian Journal of Statistics*, 41(3):387–397, 2013.

[83] X. R. Pan. *Empirical Likelihood Ratio Method for Censored Data*. Ph.D. Dissertation, University of Kentucky, 1997.

[84] X. R. Pan and M. Zhou. Empirical likelihood ratio in terms of cumulative hazard function for censored data. *Journal of Multivariate Analysis*, 80:166–188, 2002.

[85] M. I. Parzen, L. J. Wei, and Z. Ying. Simultaneous confidence intervals for the difference of two survival functions. *Scandinavian Journal of Statistics*, 24(3):309–314, 1997.

[86] H. Peng and A. Schick. An empirical likelihood approach to goodness of fit testing. *Bernoulli*, 19:954–981, 2013.

[87] S. Portnoy. Censored quantile regression. *Journal of the American Statistical Association*, 98:1001–1012, 2003.

[88] R. Prentice. Linear rank tests with right censored data. *Biometrika*, 65:167–179, 1978.

[89] G. Qin and B. Y. Jing. Empirical likelihood for Cox regression model under random censorship. *Communications in Statistics, Simulation and Computation*, 30(1):79–90, 2001.

[90] G. Qin and M. Tsao. Empirical likelihood ratio confidence interval for the trimmed mean. *Communications in Statistics, Theory and Methods*, 31:2197–2208, 2002.

[91] G. Qin, B. Yang, and N. Belinga-Hall. Empirical likelihood-based inferences for the Lorenz curve. *Annals of the Institute of Statistical Mathematics*, 65:1–21, 2013.

[92] J. Qin and J. Lawless. Empirical likelihood and general estimating equations. *Annals of Statistics*, 22:300–325, 1994.

[93] R Development Core Team. *R: A Language and Environment for Statistical Computing*. R Foundation for Statistical Computing, Vienna, Austria, 2008.

[94] J. Ren. Weighted empirical likelihood ratio confidence intervals for the mean with censored data. *Annals of the Institute of Statistical Mathematics*, 53:498–516, 2001.

[95] J. Ren. Weighted empirical likelihood in some two-sample semiparametric models with various types of censored data. *Annals of Statistics*, 36:147–166, 2008.

[96] J. Ren and M. Zhou. Full likelihood inferences in the Cox model: An empirical likelihood approach. *Annals of the Institute of Statistical Mathematics*, 63(5):1005–1018, 2011.

[97] Y. Ritov. Estimation of a linear regression model with censored data. *Annals of Statistics*, 18:303–328, 1990.

[98] A. Rotnitzky and J. M. Robins. Inverse probability weighted estimation in survival analysis. in *The Encyclopedia of Biostatistics, 2nd edition*, P. Armitage and T. Coulton, Eds. New York: Wiley, 2005.

[99] G. Satten and S. Datta. The Kaplan–Meier estimator as an inverse-probability-of-censoring weighted average. *American Statistician*, 55:207–210, 2001.

[100] S. Schennach. Bayesian exponentially tilted empirical likelihood. *Biometrika*, 92:31–46, 2005.

[101] S. Schennach. Point estimation with exponentially tilted empirical likelihood. *Annals of Statistics*, 35:634–672, 2007.

[102] A. Schick. Empirical likelihood with martingale differences. *Preprint*, 2014.

[103] J. Shen and S. He. Empirical likelihood for the difference of two survival functions under right censorship. *Statistics and Probability Letters*, 76:169–181, 2006.

[104] C. Srinivasan and M. Zhou. Linear regression with censoring. *Journal of Multivariate Analysis*, 49:179–201, 1994.

[105] C. Stein. Efficient nonparametric testing and estimation. *Proc. Third Berkeley Symp. on Math. Statist. and Prob., Vol. 1*, pages 187–195, 1956.

[106] W. Stute. Distributional convergence under random censorship when covariables are present. *Scandinavian Journal of Statistics*, 23:461–471, 1996.

[107] W. Stute. The jackknife estimate of variance of a Kaplan–Meier integral. *Annals of Statistics*, 24:2679–2704, 1996.

[108] W. Stute. Nonlinear censored regression. *Statistica Sinica*, 9:1089–1102, 1999.

[109] W. Stute and J. Wang. The jackknife estimate of a Kaplan–Meier integral. *Biometrika*, 81:602–606, 1994.

[110] X. Sun, P. Peng, and D. Tu. Phase II cancer clinical trials with a one-sample log-rank test and its corrections based on the Edgeworth expansion. *Contemporary Clinical Trials*, 32:108–113, 2011.

[111] T. Therneau and P. Grambsch. *Modeling Survival Data: Extending the Cox Model*. Springer, 2000.

[112] D. R. Thomas and G. L. Grunkemeier. Confidence interval estimation of survival probabilities for censored data. *Journal of the American Statistical Association*, 70(352):865–871, 1975.

[113] G. Tripathi. A matrix extension of the Cauchy–Schwarz inequality. *Economics Letters*, 63:1–3, 1999.

[114] M. Tsao and C. Wu. Empirical likelihood inference for a common mean in the presence of heteroscedasticity. *Canadian Journal of Statistics*, 34:45–59, 2006.

[115] A. Tsiatis. A nonidentifiability aspect of the problem of competing risks. *Proceedings of the National Academy of Sciences*, 72:20–22, 1975.

[116] A. Tsiatis. A large sample study of Cox's regression model. *Annals of Statistics*, 9(1):93–108, 1981.

[117] A. Tsiatis. Estimating regression parameters using linear rank tests for censored data. *Annals of Statistics*, 18:354–372, 1990.

[118] B. W. Turnbull. The empirical distribution function with arbitrarily grouped, censored and truncated data. *Journal of the Royal Statistical Society. Series B (Methodological)*, pages 290–295, 1976.

[119] M. J. van der Laan and J. M. Robins. *Unified Methods for Censored Longitudinal Data and Causality*. Springer Verlag: New York, 2003.

[120] M. C. A. van Zuijlen. Properties of the empirical distribution function for independent non-identically distributed random vectors. *Annals of Probability*, 10:108–123, 1982.

[121] M. Velina and J. Valeinis. Empirical likelihood-based robust inference for trimmed means. *Preprint*, 2013.

[122] Q. H. Wang and B. Y. Jing. Empirical likelihood for a class of functionals of survival distribution with censored data. *Annals of the Institute of Statistical Mathematics*, 53(3):517–527, 2001.

[123] G. Wei and D. Schaubel. Estimating cumulative treatment effects in the presence of nonproportional hazards. *Biometrics*, 64(3):724–732, 2008.

[124] L. J. Wei, Z. Ying, and D. Y. Lin. Linear regression analysis of censored survival data based on rank tests. *Biometrika*, 77:845–851, 1990.

[125] R. Woolson. Rank test and a one-sample logrank test for comparing observed survival data to a standard population. *Biometrics*, 37:687–696, 1981.

[126] C. Wu. Combining information from multiple surveys through empirical likelihood method. *Canadian Journal of Statistics*, 32:15–26, 2004.

[127] J. Wu. A new one-sample log-rank test. *Journal of Biometrics and Biostatistics*, 5:210, 2014.

[128] D. Yang and D. S. Small. An R package and a study of methods for computing empirical likelihood. *Journal of Statistical Computing and Simulation*, 41:1–10, 2012.

[129] S. Yang and R. Prentice. Semiparametric analysis of short-term and long-term hazard ratios with two-sample survival data. *Biometrika*, 92:1–17, 2005.

[130] Z. Ying. A large sample study of rank estimation for censored regression data. *Annals of Statistics*, 21:76–99, 1993.

[131] Z. Ying, S. Jung, and L. J. Wei. Survival analysis with median regression models. *Journal of the American Statistical Association*, 90(429):178–184, 1995.

[132] M. Zhang and J. Klein. Confidence bands for the difference of two survival curves under proportional hazards model. *Lifetime Data Analysis*, 7(3):243–254, 2001.

[133] B. Zhong and J. N. K. Rao. Empirical likelihood inference under stratified random sampling using auxiliary population information. *Biometrika*, 87:929–938, 2000.

[134] M. Zhou. Some properties of the Kaplan–Meier estimator for independent non-identically distributed random variables. *Annals of Statistics*, 19:2266–2274, 1991.

[135] M. Zhou. M-estimation in censored linear models. *Biometrka*, 79:837–841, 1992.

[136] M. Zhou. Understanding the Cox regression models with time-change covariates. *American Statistician*, 55:153–155, 2001.

[137] M. Zhou. Empirical likelihood analysis of the rank estimator for the censored accelerated failure time model. *Biometrika*, 92:492–498, 2005.

[138] M. Zhou. Empirical likelihood ratio with arbitrarily censored/truncated data by EM algorithm. *Journal of Computational and Graphical Statistics*, 14(3):643–656, 2005.

[139] M. Zhou. The Cox proportional hazards model with partially known baseline. In *Random Walk, Sequential Analysis and Related Topics,* Chao Agnes Hsiung, Zhiliang Ying and Cun-Hui Zhang, Eds.; World Scientific Publishing, pages 215–232, 2006.

[140] M. Zhou and J. Jeong. Empirical likelihood test for mean and median residual life times. *Statistics in Medicine*, 30:152–159, 2011.

[141] M. Zhou, M. Kim, and A. Bathke. Empirical likelihood analysis for the heteroscedastic accelerated failure time model. *Statistica Sinica*, 22:295–316, 2012.

[142] M. Zhou and G. Li. Empirical likelihood analysis of the Buckley–James estimator. *Journal of Multivariate Analysis*, 99(4):649–664, 2008.

[143] M. Zhou and Y. Yang. A recursive formula for the Kaplan–Meier estimator with mean constraints and its application to empirical likelihood. *Computational Statistics*, 2015.

[144] H. Zhu. *Smoothed Empirical Likelihood for Quantiles and Some Variations/Extension of Empirical Likelihood for Buckley–James Estimator.* Ph.D. Dissertation, University of Kentucky, 2007.

[145] S. Zhu. *Empirical Likelihood Confidence Band.* Ph.D. Dissertation, University of Kentucky, 2015.

[146] S. Zhu, M. Zhou, and S. Wei. Empirical likelihood inference on survival functions under proportional hazards model. *Journal of Biometrics and Biostatistics*, 5:206, 2014.

[147] S. Zhu, M. Zhou, and Y. Yang. A note on the empirical likelihood confidence band for hazards ratio with covariate adjustment. *Biometrics*, 2015.

Index

Accelerated failure time model, 119
advanced time, 73
advanced time transformation, 63

Buckley–James estimator, 121, 152

censored data, 1
central limit theorem, 32
confidence band, 187
confidence interval, 163
correlation model, 120
counting process, 56
Cox proportional hazards model, 1, 91
cross hazards, 42
cumulative hazard function, 2

EM algorithm, 146
empirical distribution, 12
empirical likelihood, 1, 12

feasible region, 25

Gehan estimator, 44
Gehan test, 38
generalized Lorenz curve, 156
Gini index, 156
Greenwood, 8

hazard, 23
hazard function, 2

intermediate parameters, 154

jackknife, 139

Kaplan–Meier, 1

least favorable distribution, 63
log rank estimator, 44

log rank test, 37
Lorenz curve, 156

martingale, 58
martingale difference, 15
matrix Cauchy–Schwarz inequality, 71
maximum empirical likelihood estimator, 42
maximum likelihood estimator, 5
median regression, 133
median residual lifetime, 73

Nelson–Aalen, 7, 24

optimal confidence regions, 173
Overdetermined estimating equations, 46

piecewise exponential, 9
piecewise exponential model, 6
plug-in EL, 172
Poisson process, 56
predictable function, 37
profile, 154
proportional hazards, 41
pseudo EL, 172

quantile, 183

ratio of hazards, 166
recursive algorithm, 147
regression model, 120

scale, 175
score test, 177
self-consistency, 73
sequential quadratic programming, 145
short-term/long-term hazard ratio model, 109
smoothing, 183

Milton Keynes UK
Ingram Content Group UK Ltd.
UKHW040059071024
449327UK00019B/666